Nursing Homes

Nursing Homes
getting good care there

Sarah Greene Burger
Virginia Fraser
Sara Hunt
Barbara Frank

Second Edition

A Consumer Action Manual Prepared by
The National Citizens' Coalition for Nursing Home Reform

Impact **Publishers,® Inc.**
ATASCADERO, CALIFORNIA

ATTENTION ORGANIZATIONS AND CORPORATIONS:
This book is available at quantity discounts on bulk purchases for educational, business, or sales promotional use. For further information, please contact Impact Publishers, P.O. Box 6016, Atascadero, CA 93423-6016, Phone: 1-800-246-7228, e-mail: sales@impactpublishers.com

Library of Congress Cataloging-in-Publication Data

Nursing homes: getting good care there / Sarah Greene Burger ... [et al.] – 2nd ed.
    p. cm.
    "A consumer action manual prepared by the National Citizens' Coalition for Nursing Home Reform."
    Includes index.
    ISBN 1-886230-43-9
        1. Nursing home care--United States. 2. Nursing homes--Evaluation.
    I. Burger, Sarah. II. National Citizens' Coalition for Nursing Home Reform.

RA997 .N897 2001
362.1'6'0973--dc21   2001046334

Publisher's Note
This publication is designed to provide accurate and authoritative information in regard to the subject matter covered. It is sold with the understanding that the publisher is not engaged in rendering psychological, legal, financial, or other professional services. If expert assistance or counseling is needed, the services of a competent professional should be sought.

Impact Publishers and colophon are registered trademarks of Impact Publishers, Inc.

Cover design by Sharon Schnare, San Luis Obispo, California.
Printed in the United States of America on acid-free paper,
Published by **Impact ✎ Publishers, Inc.**
POST OFFICE BOX 6016
ATASCADERO, CALIFORNIA 93423-6016
www.impactpublishers.com

Contents

Preface

VIRTUALLY EVERY DECISION TO SELECT A NURSING HOME, personally or by the family, is crisis-driven. People are desperate and often unable or incapable of spending the time and attention needed to find the best possible facility. Even those who are wary about nursing homes have to trust that they have chosen the best possible place for themselves or their loved one. Yet, families *should* be able to have faith in their decision, for nursing home care is guided and governed by public laws, regulations and standards that hold great promise. Moreover, America's national nursing home reform law (Public Law 100-203 in the *Social Security Act)* pledges specifically that *each resident* who lives in a nursing home is to receive quality of care, be afforded quality of life, and have specific rights and privileges maintained.

Fortunately, many people do select a nursing home that is meeting its contractual obligations so specifically laid out in law. Out of America's 17,000 nursing homes, in every state there are many nursing homes that strive daily to maintain public standards. Increasingly, many go even further and adopt and apply pioneering approaches that result in high quality care that is resident-directed and engages families and others in positive ways.

Distressingly, far too many nursing homes still fail to meet public standards. They provide, at best, mediocre care. Moreover, far too many fail miserably, and many residents in these facilities suffer needlessly from neglect and even abusive care. That is why the National Citizens' Coalition for Nursing Home Reform (NCCNHR) fought so long for this law in 1987. These persistent problems are why the national reform law directs state governments to inspect facilities and enforce standards.

Still, despite what the law directs, there are serious flaws in many state and federal enforcement programs. Too often, deficiencies go undetected and standards unenforced. In addition to the enforcement program another safety net is the national long-term care ombudsmen programs, prescribed in the federal *Older Americans Act in 1978*. Every state has established an ombudsman program. Ombudsmen, both paid and volunteers, visit facilities, listen to residents, help resolve their problems, and, with the resident's permission, refer serious complaints to the survey and inspection agency. Ombudsmen programs strive to provide education about nursing home care and the rights of residents. The work of the program is critical to help monitor nursing homes, as well as board and care, assisted living and other long-term care settings. In spite of this program's importance to residents and families, ombudsmen are often short on funds, time and volunteers to meet the critical needs.

NCCNHR and other advocacy groups around the country advocate daily for quality of life and care for residents in nursing homes. Our advocacy takes many forms. We monitor government regulatory activities and continually push for stronger enforcement of existing laws. We participate in government meetings to help drive decisions that are centered on the needs of the vulnerable, ill, and disabled individuals who require services. We provide public education and training for advocates and ombudsmen. We assist and respond to the media when it focuses on substandard nursing home care. Whenever possible, we work in collaboration with groups of health care professionals, providers and research scientists to advance the strongest possible standards and protections for residents. For example, because of the serious shortage of staff in nursing homes, we developed a minimum staffing standard that is supported by many organizations. And, we assist and work with family members, particularly in the development of strong, effective family councils.

Families are a critical component of the nursing home system of care. There is an essential role for family members in helping to obtain and maintain the quality of care and life for residents prescribed by law. This book guides families in achieving good care for residents in nursing homes.

The authors of *Nursing Homes: Getting Good Care There* are advocates, experienced professionals, who represent over one hundred years of caring, concern, advocacy and knowledge about the day-to-day life of residents living in nursing homes. Three (Frank, Fraser, and Hunt) have served as state long-term care ombudsmen. One (Burger) is a nurse who has worked in nursing homes, a long-time advocate, and former NCCNHR executive director. Frank and Hunt have also worked directly for NCCNHR providing valuable work in policy development, advocacy and training. In this book , so generously donated to our organization, the authors provide a wealth of insights, information, and encouragement to help residents, family members, resident and family councils be advocates for change. Because it carefully describes the intent of the reform law and offers valuable ideas for care giving, the book will also be useful for nursing home staff and management and other professionals working to achieve quality care for residents.

NCCNHR is confident that your concerns about getting good nursing home care will be addressed in the pages that follow. You will be rewarded with improved care as you boldly and consistently apply the advocacy information and techniques provided in this valuable consumer guide. We hope that you will also become a part of NCCNHR's advocacy network by joining our organization, especially in its work to achieve our proposed standard for increased nursing home staffing. It will take all of us, advocates, ombudsmen, regulators, caring nursing home staff, health care professionals, *and you* to see that *each resident* receives the protection, services and benefits promised by law. It is the least we should expect for our elders and citizens with disabilities who need the care nursing homes are responsible for providing.

By Elma L. Holder, Founder
The National Citizens' Coalition for Nursing Home Reform

Introduction

Help me. Please help me!

Rose heard the cry as she hurried down the corridor toward her mother's room. She recognized her mother's voice, and noted that none of the busy nursing home staff were responding to the pleas. It wasn't the first time. Her mother had frequently complained of being ignored in recent weeks. Staff responded that "She calls out all the time! We can't run into her room every five minutes!" Rose found her mother slumped down in her seat, pulling at the tray top of her wheelchair. Rose approached her mother, bending down and gently touching one arm. Her mother turned her face toward the caring voice that asked, "How can I help you, Mom?"

If someone you love lives in a nursing home, this book can help you be an effective advocate for better care. You can make a difference in the attention and services your relative receives. We've worked with thousands of families and friends of residents across the country, and we've seen how their constructive, informed involvement can improve life for their loved ones.

This book is a guide to help you advocate for your mother, father, brother, sister, grandfather, grandmother, aunt, uncle, friend, neighbor — anyone you care about who lives in a nursing home. With this book as your resource, you'll know what concerns are legitimate and what you can do about them. If you know how to ask the right questions, you can channel your concern into effective advocacy for better care. By speaking up you may be able to work out your concerns with the staff.

Does the idea of being an "advocate" sound a little uncomfortable? Don't be put off. We're simply encouraging you to be the person who — as the dictionary tells us — "pleads the cause" or "speaks out in support" of your loved one. It's not an easy job, but when you see the results, we're convinced you'll agree that it's worth every bit of energy it takes.

Negotiating with the staff of a nursing home can seem intimidating and overwhelming. Problems can be widespread and enormous, and it can seem that you're alone against "the system." You're not. There are advocates in every state and most localities — called *ombudsmen* — available to assist you. They can advise you about your rights and the nursing home's responsibilities. They'll help you identify and discuss the changes you would like to see. Some states also have citizen advocacy groups that can help you.

This book tells about good care practices, about resident's rights and staff's responsibilities. It explains the laws and government regulations that give you the power to get good care.

This is a time of change in nursing home care! Federal and state laws offer strong consumer protection and have begun raising the standard of care. The federal Nursing Home Reform Law (1987) has brought about substantial improvements in the lives of residents. Health care professionals have learned more about good care practices. Consumers are more knowledgeable and willing to speak up.

All these forces — better laws, better professional standards of practice, more consumer involvement — have led to improvements in conditions in many nursing homes. Now, as we face changes in our health care delivery system, you can make sure those improvements benefit the one you love.

It's All "Relative"
Maybe you picked up this book because you have a relative in a nursing home; perhaps it's a close friend. Or you may be a conscientious nursing home staff member who'd like to enhance your caregiving skills. Or maybe you just want to know more about good care in nursing homes.

In this book, we use the term "relative" to identify the resident you care about. Most advocates *are* relatives, so the term helps to simplify our presentation. Even if you're not related, however, we're sure you'll find the information useful!

You Can Advocate for Better Care

Having someone you love move into a nursing home can be a devastating experience. Tens of thousands of families and friends struggle every year through the decision to turn to a nursing home for care. It's difficult to accept that a relative can no longer take care of herself, and that you can't take care of her. It is hard to see someone you love leave her home and lose her independence. Becoming a protector to your parent, sibling or friend, is unsettling. And especially so if the person is one who has cared for you in earlier years; it's not easy to see the roles reversed.

Your experiences and fears are normal and appropriate. Don't be afraid to seek advice and support as you go through this stressful time.

Working with the Staff

Consumers expect more from nursing homes these days, and families are working cooperatively with staff to insure more personalized care. The few weeks after admission are a crucial time when you can help the staff learn how to make a new resident, your relative, feel at home.

Giving staff a view of your relative as the valued person he is helps them see beyond the daily caregiving tasks to your relative as an individual. Bigger problems often begin over little matters about daily life routine. When nursing home staff are driven by tasks, rules, and institutional regimens, the needs of individual residents can be left behind.

But it needn't be that way. Thanks to stronger laws, effective advocacy, and increasing professionalism in health care delivery, the *home* in nursing home is becoming a reality in many places. Staff are asking what they can do as health professionals to give care and comfort to each resident as an individual. And everyone benefits. When homes revolve around residents, they operate more efficiently and cost-effectively. Individualized care is good for residents and their families, for staff, and for the nursing home. Instead of your fears about the need for nursing home care, you can feel the relief of knowing that kind, caring, skilled professionals have provided the support and security your relative needs at this difficult time in her life.

You can help make it happen.

Who's Who On the Staff?

You might be wondering whom you should see if you have questions or concerns. Since the *certified nurse assistants (CNA's)* are closest to your relative, you can ask them how things are going. Talk with them about your relative's preferences. The caregiving connection between CNA's and residents is at the heart of quality care.

If you have clinical questions or need someone who can make decisions about care, talk with a nurse (RN or LPN/LVN). Many times your questions can be answered by the nurse in charge of the unit where your relative lives. Although nursing homes use different titles for positions, this person will usually be called the *charge nurse,* the *head nurse, team leader,* or *supervisor.* If you need to speak to the person in charge of all nursing services, you'll need to see the *director of nursing.* To ask for a care plan meeting, begin by talking with the charge nurse. Of course there usually are individuals responsible for each area of a nursing home such as housekeeping, dietary, social services, and activities. You'll want to talk with them about questions and concerns related to their specialties. Don't be reluctant to ask questions of staff!

Nationwide Standards of Care

Personalized care in a place that "feels like home" is possible mainly because of changes in practice that are supported by the Nursing Home Reform Law. This law was passed by the U.S. Congress in 1987 because of serious concerns about problems in nursing homes.

In developing the law, Congress relied on *Improving the Quality of Care in Nursing Homes,* a landmark report in 1986 by the Institute of Medicine, which called for a major overhaul of government oversight of nursing homes. The report recommended changes in federal government regulations, improved procedures for inspection of nursing homes, and strengthened enforcement of the laws. The report also highlighted the important role that advocacy and community involvement play in the effort to improve care.

The 1987 law set new standards for every nursing home that participates in Medicare or Medicaid, a state funded payment program. If your relative lives in a facility that doesn't participate in either of these programs, you'll need to check your state's laws for specific information on requirements for care. The principles embedded in the Nursing Home Reform Law have raised the standard of quality nursing home care. The care guidelines and good practice tips in this book have become the accepted standard of practice among health care professionals. These guidelines and tips are also useful in any long term care setting, even if an individual is receiving care in her own home.

The central theme of the new standards is that nursing homes must provide services in a way that helps each person live to her fullest potential — physically, mentally, and emotionally.

Be Involved!

Your involvement and advocacy can improve your relative's care and life in the home. To be involved you must be informed about residents' rights, good models of care, the laws that govern nursing home practice, and programs and agencies in your state to help residents and families. *This book has the information you need.* To prepare you for some situations you may encounter, it's filled with real-life examples and everyday solutions.

Don't Accept the Status Quo

As you set out to advocate for good care, the most important thing to know is that change for the better is possible: *You don't have to accept the status quo!* Services for residents can improve when consumers ask for better care and professionals learn more about new ways to address situations. Speaking up for your relative can make things better. Start by *expecting* good care. Learn more about what nursing homes are required to do. Become an effective advocate for the person you love. This book tells you how.

About the Book

We encourage you to *use this book however it is most helpful to you.* You might choose to turn immediately to a chapter that talks about a topic of interest to you. The book is organized so you don't have to read it in order. (The chapter sequence seems logical to us, but what matters is how it works for you!) Read it as you need information.

Chapter 1 introduces you to the individual experience of entering a nursing home. It discusses residents' struggle to retain individuality within an institutional routine. It also introduces you to new approaches to care that put the individual first. This chapter tells you how to help your relative *from day one.*

Chapter 2 focuses on *residents'* rights. Federal and state laws affirm residents' rights to make choices about their lives, to exercise control over their care and treatment, and to have information about what is happening to them. The chapter is packed with examples, including such issues as financial affairs, the right to question treatment, and rights regarding transfer or relocation.

Chapter 3 gives information about planning your relative's care based on an assessment. You'll learn what the nursing home needs to ask about your relative in the assessment process and how that assessment information forms the basis of a care plan. Read this chapter to find out how your relative and you can help with the all-important process of *assessment and care planning.*

Chapter 4 covers the *seven most common problems in care.* Standards for good care are discussed so you'll know what should be done for your relative. You'll learn about *quality of care* and what this means in nursing homes. What should you expect the nursing home to do to prevent incontinence, dehydration, malnutrition, skin breakdown, contractures, depression, and other avoidable conditions? You'll find out what warning signs to look for, questions to ask, and when and how to intervene.

Chapter 5 describes the dangers of *physical and chemical restraints.* If you think restraints are the only way to address such behavioral symptoms as wandering and agitation, read this chapter. Restraints do not resolve these problems, they only make matters worse! We explain why, and let you know what you can do about it.

Chapter 6 is about the *quality of life* in a nursing home. Medical care is only half the story; it's the quality of a person's life in the home that has the biggest impact on her well-being. Nursing home professionals have learned a lot about how to make facilities feel more like "home." This chapter includes suggestions for helping staff adjust the daily routine to your relative's life-long habits and personal preferences.

Chapter 7 is a guide to *problem-solving.* Once you have the tools described in chapters 2-6, you can use chapter 7 to help with specific concerns. You may choose to talk personally with the administrative staff of the nursing home, or you may want to work with other families through a family council. Outside assistance is also available. You'll learn where to go for more help if needed.

Chapter 8 puts the nursing home system in context. Why are some homes better than others? How do money, politics and leadership affect nursing home care? You'll find answers to these questions, and a compelling example of how good leadership can ensure good care. And, you'll be encouraged to stay involved in working for better care for the people you love.

A Note About Short-Term Residence — "Sub-Acute Care" and Other Settings

Many people now go to nursing homes for short-term rehabilitation (called "sub-acute care") after a hospitalization. These stays are usually 21 to 90 days. This can be a positive opportunity to receive needed therapy before returning home, but some consumer concerns may arise, particularly if your relative needs more rehabilitative services after the Medicare benefits end. *The material discussed in this book applies to short-term stays as well!* Review chapters 2, 3, 4, and 5. The information about good care (chapters 4 and 5) also applies regardless of the place of residence such as assisted living or in the person's own home.

You Can Make a Difference!

We think you'll find this book helpful as you seek "good care there." Your constructive intervention can turn a nursing home situation around for your relative. As a bonus, other residents may also benefit from your work. Remember, you're not alone in your efforts! There are nearly 1.5 million nursing home residents in the U.S, and tens of thousands of families share your questions and concerns.

Learn your rights. Learn about good care. Use that information to speak up. Don't give up. Expect good care and voice your concerns. It's the only way things will get better. You can make a difference!

Chapter 1

Individualized Care

You haven't lived til you've gone to the toilet on somebody else's schedule!"
— told by a nursing home resident to Carter Williams

Y OU'LL RECALL THIS SCENE FROM THE INTRODUCTION: "Help me... please help me," Rose heard as she hurried to her mother's room. She found her in distress.

"Help me, please," her mother begged. "I've dropped my shoe and I can't reach it. And now I can't get back up."

Rose asked an aide for help, and together they straightened her mother in the chair. As her mother calmed down, they began their daily visit.

On the way home that evening, Rose resolved to talk with the staff about her concerns, as she had on earlier occasions, with help from the local long-term care ombudsman. The staff had responded with some important changes in their approach to her mother's care. Mrs. Beck had lived at the home for six months. Her Alzheimer's disease had progressed rapidly since her admission, and she often acted upset. She had hit staff members, and even spit a time or two — very unlike her mother. Staff confined her to her geri-chair (a wheelchair with a tray in front) for "safety."

Life Before the Nursing Home

Rose recalled telling the ombudsman about her mother's typical day at home. "Mother loved to stay up late with a good book, a warm blanket, and a hot glass of milk. She'd often have a hot bath first and then sit in her favorite chair till one in the morning, reading. She was a late riser, usually not getting up until ten or so. She wasn't much for conversation or activity in the morning. Oh, and her favorite breakfast was a bowl of ice cream!"

Life in the Nursing Home

Rose compared this pattern with life for Mrs. Beck at the nursing home. Here the routine was to get up at 7, and to be ready for a full breakfast at 8. Next came the procession to the shower so everyone could be dressed and presentable before lunch. Sure enough, incident upon incident documented by staff had occurred in the morning, when Mrs. Beck was too sleepy to be handled and too confused to say "no" in words. So she struck out and was labeled a "behavior problem." Staff, already overworked, didn't have enough time to respond each time she called out for help.

The situation was easily resolved by adapting the daily routine to her mother's needs. The Activities Director arranged for large-print books, the Charge Nurse adjusted the schedule for bathing and personal care, and the Social Worker helped other staff learn how to defuse situations when Mrs. Back became upset. "But now here we are again," Rose thought. "Time for another meeting with the staff. We need to get this new situation straightened out." She saw that the aides were so busy "getting the job done" that they had become dulled to such frequent cries for assistance.

Attention to Individuals

You too may have heard someone crying out for help as you visited a nursing home. Perhaps you, like Rose, were told, "Oh, she does that all the time. You can just ignore her." Too often staff are so strained that they draw a mental curtain to tune out the cries.

As a family member, you can talk with staff about ways to respond to your relative that can be soothing for her and can provide the help and human contact she needs.

Hesitant? Of course. It's natural to feel unsure of yourself in such a situation. The staff are working hard, often rushing from one crisis to another without time to question what they're doing. That's why it's so important to call staff attention to situations that they no longer notice. Although staff may be working hard, good care requires that they have the time to respond to residents' pleas for assistance.

Quality care involves caring for the resident's human spirit as well as her physical health. Nurses, doctors and other health care workers have come to recognize that some of their old approaches to care — restraints, for example — actually do more harm than good. For a long time, nursing homes and state regulatory agencies focused more on immediate efforts to provide "safety," not realizing that short term, stop gap, "safety" measures often have long term negative effects on residents' physical and emotional well-being.

— Quality care involves caring for the resident's human spirit as well as her physical health. —

What Would You Want if You Were in a Nursing Home?

To examine what good care is, it's important to think about what you would want if you lived in a nursing home. For most people, it's a difficult scene to imagine.

Why? Is the idea of being so sick troubling? Is it fear of dying? Certainly these feelings are natural. But there's something even more unsettling about imagining yourself in a nursing home: *the fear of losing control or independence.* Most people are frightened at the thought of losing their independence as they grow older. Yet some physical and mental decline and increased dependency are inevitable with age.

You may spend part of your own life in a nursing home, so when you think about what nursing homes should be like, pay attention to your own needs and preferences. Doing so will help you better understand what people living in nursing homes are feeling.

Begin by asking yourself, "What if I were to enter a nursing home today? What would I want a nursing home to be like to feel okay about living there?"

Does your image of an acceptable nursing home include being treated with dignity, respect, recognition of your individuality? Would you expect compassion, privacy, choice over aspects of daily life in the nursing home? If so, you share a lot in common with thousands of others across the country who have answered this question.

What Do Residents Say?

As part of a national study, the National Citizens' Coalition for Nursing Home Reform (NCCNHR) asked residents about their views on quality care. Groups of residents in nursing homes in fifteen cities across the United States gave their definition of quality care. The primary factors they listed were:

- treatment with dignity and respect;
- self-determination and the opportunity to make choices about their daily lives; and
- kind, caring staff who regarded them as individuals.

In the years since the study was conducted in 1985, the National Citizens' Coalition has posed the same question — "How would you define quality care if you lived in a nursing home?" — to advocates, family members, nursing home staff and government officials throughout the country. Consistently, respondents say they want to have their individuality

> *—The basic human need to continue "being who I am" is perhaps the most important need of anyone living in a nursing home. —*

supported and respected. The basic human need to continue "being who I am" is perhaps the most important need of anyone living in a nursing home.

You might be surprised to learn that *supporting* individuality for each resident has become the standard of care.

In the past, many nursing homes did too little to truly support individuality among residents. Throughout this book, you'll discover how and why this is changing, how staff are helping residents feel more at home. To better appreciate what moving into a nursing home is like from a resident's perspective, read on!

From Home to... Homeless?

The losses most people experience as they go from their own homes into nursing homes are enormous. It's traumatic to make the transition to nursing home life. There are lots of losses that bring about such a move. There are also losses that come because of the move.

Increasing mental and/or physical frailty forces a person to leave the last vestiges of independence and turn to a nursing home — possibly for the rest of his life.

Think about the word "home." What does it mean to you? Do you have warm feelings and images? Are you thinking about family? Security? A place where you can kick your shoes off and be yourself?

Think about how you feel as a guest in someone else's home. Remember what it's like when it's not your kitchen? Not your bathroom? Not your special chair in the living room? Do you breathe a sigh of relief at the thought of the trip's end and your return home?

Multiply that feeling by 365 days a year, and you'll sense the perpetual anxiety and tension — as a permanent "guest" — felt by most nursing home residents. In 1990 nurse Judith Carboni* found a correlation between the experience of living in a nursing home and the experience of homelessness. All the ways that *home* represents connection, safety, security and privacy are not easily available to nursing home residents. Home is an important link to identity — connection to people, places, events in our lives. Look around your home and see all the reminders you've accumulated.

Nursing home residents experience disconnection and loss of identity. Residents may try to cling in their minds to their own identities and their pasts. But, instead of feeling secure, they feel anxious; instead of privacy they feel constantly exposed and vulnerable.

One major loss of the feeling of home is loss of daily routine. We all develop ways of living that provide comfort and help us function — our ways of handling stress, our social outlets, our interests and our pursuits. It could be talking with a friend, watching sports, listening to the radio, working on a hobby, gardening, reading... Unfortunately, these patterns of living have often been the first things people have been expected to sacrifice when entering a nursing home. Under current standards, however, nursing homes are now expected to support each resident's life patterns. (Reading chapter 2 on residents' rights and chapter 6 on quality of life will show you how things can change.)

— *"You haven't lived 'til you've gone to the toilet on somebody else's schedule!"* —

"You haven't lived 'til you've gone to the toilet on somebody else's schedule!" That's how one elderly resident described her life in a nursing home to social worker Carter Williams. Residents' daily

---

*Carboni, Judith (1990). "Homelessness Among The Institutionalized Elderly." *Journal of Gerontological Nursing*, 16 (7) 32-37.

needs become staff tasks. Take a few moments to consider — from a resident's perspective — the basic routine of bathing.

Joanne Rader*, a nurse in Oregon, studied bathing in nursing homes for people with dementia. To begin her research, Rader decided to be given a shower as residents are. Her staff was taken aback by her request. "Oh my, you're brave!" they said. They believed showering her would feel awkward and embarrassing. In fact, it did, even though staff used a skillful and caring manner.

Nurse Rader experienced being wheeled through the hallway with a sheet wrapped around her, then hoisted and handled, sprayed by gushing water, all the time surrounded by cold metal. Throughout, she had the feeling of being exposed and cold and embarrassed. No wonder people with dementia are apt to become agitated during a bath, she mused. Their agitation probably is not so much an inevitable part of nursing home life as it is a predictable reaction to a stressful experience!

Clinicians find that agitation can be soothed if nursing homes are less like institutions and more like home. Nursing homes can be more home-like by respecting residents' individuality. Home routines can be adapted to accommodate individuals, rather than asking people to fit into institutional schedules for toileting and eating and bathing — for the convenience of staff.

— Agitation can be soothed if nursing homes are less like institutions and more like home. —

Putting the "Home" Back Into Nursing Home

The 1987 Nursing Home Reform Law, often referred to as "OBRA '87" because it was part of that year's federal Omnibus Budget Reconciliation Act, motivated many nursing homes to rethink their approaches to care. Born from ardent concerns and grassroots action by consumers and pioneering health care professionals, the law helped turn the concept of caregiving around. In the days before the law, residents were told to "adjust" to the nursing home's daily routines. Now the law asks nursing home staff to adjust to residents' daily routines.

— Facilities save money by giving good care! —

---

*Rader, Joanne (1995). "Individualized Approaches to Care." Norwich, CT: *Breaking the Bonds Conference*, June 21.

Although we are a long way from completing this change in thinking but we have made progress. Forward thinking nursing home staff have always approached care in a way that supports individuality. As laws have changed and staff see the benefits of responding to residents' individual needs, many practitioners are learning new approaches to care.

☞   TIP: Administrators of nursing homes who have decided to change routines and accommodate individuals have found they can do so with the same staff and resources and find that it is even more cost effective to do so. The bottom line: *facilities save money by giving good care!* This was documented by Catherine Hawes of the Research Triangle Institute in 1995.*
     As professional staff have begun to change practice, there has been an overall improvement — nationwide — in residents' physical and mental functioning. However, nursing homes need enough staff so that staff can take the time to get to know residents as individuals. Working regularly with the same residents also helps staff individualize care.

As consumers begin expecting nursing homes to act differently and supporting nursing homes in new ways of working, change will continue.

The federal law brought a new philosophy based on two very important requirements: *Quality of Care* and *Quality of Life.*

• **Quality of Care** means nursing home residents should get better whenever possible, should maintain the highest possible level of physical, mental, and psychosocial functioning, and at the very least, should not get worse because of the care received from the nursing home.

— Residents should not get worse unless their decline is medically unavoidable. —

The *quality of care* requirements include activities of daily living, such as eating, bathing, dressing and walking. They also involve such matters as skin condition, continence, range of motion and psychosocial well-being. In all these areas, *residents should not get worse unless their decline is medically unavoidable.* This means that a

---

*Hawes, Catherine (1995). Statement for the *Forum on Republican Medicaid Proposals to Repeal Access to Affordable Quality Nursing Care.* Washington, DC: Democratic Policy Committee (Senators Byron Dorgan, Edward Kennedy, David Pryor, Paul Sarbanes), October 6.

resident who could walk when he entered a nursing home should still be able to walk now, unless suffering a progressive disease that makes it increasingly impossible to walk, or experiencing a new debilitating problem, such as a stroke.

Too often, family members think, or are told, that a resident's decline is the inevitable effect of old age. This may not be true. While some conditions develop as people age and face illnesses, proper nursing and medical interventions can usually stop or slow the decline. Therapeutic and preventive services *do* make a difference. Older people *can* regain their mobility and function after a stroke, a fracture, or other health trauma.

When residents don't get enough exercise or food that's appealing to them, or assistance to continue activities that interest them, they decline. Such declines aren't a natural result of their medical condition, they are the result of *improper care*. They are avoidable, in some cases reversible. (More about quality of care in chapter 4.)

• **Quality of Life,** as defined in the law, means the nursing home must make reasonable accommodation for the individual needs and preferences of residents. Residents have the right to make choices about their daily schedule, health care, activities and other aspects of life in the nursing home that are meaningful and significant to them.

Just as residents should not get worse physically because of the care they receive, so they should not decline emotionally because of life in the nursing home. In her study, nurse Carboni (footnote, page 12) found that residents responded to a sense of homelessness by retreating into psychic despair, losing touch with the painful present, and exhibiting confusion and withdrawal. The loss of reasoning ability, depression, or other confusion that many residents already experience worsens their sense of homelessness.

The typical effects of depression are social withdrawal, loss of appetite, loss of sleep, confusion, weakness — many of the conditions typically found among nursing home residents. But it's important to remember that — as happens with poor quality of care — such declines don't always result from a resident's medical condition. Rather, they are a resident's natural reaction to losing a sense of self. These reactions, too, are avoidable, reversible. Attending to a resident's individual needs and making adjustments so she feels at home can help restore emotional well-being. (Read chapter 6 to learn about supporting quality of life for your relative.)

Assessment and Care Planning

The main vehicle you have to help your relative is the process of *assessment and care planning*, in which you'll participate in care decisions and helping the home support your relative's preferred life patterns.

Nursing homes must conduct an assessment of each resident. This evaluation is the basis for planning that individual's care. Just as it's necessary to look at a map to plan your route before you head out on a trip, assessment and care planning are meant to give staff direction in working with each resident. (You'll learn more about assessment and care planning in chapter 3.)

Good care planning and assessment can improve nursing home services. That's good practice, and that's the standard of care throughout the nation.

How Are the Standards Enforced... Or Are They?

You might be wondering why you don't see more personalization of care in nursing homes if this is the standard. Nursing homes are still learning how to do things differently, and consumers are still learning to expect better care. Low-staffing makes it difficult for nursing homes to provide the quality care required of them.

The government enforces the quality care standards through regular inspections, called *surveys*, to determine how well each nursing home meets the requirements. Surveyors observe care and ask residents and families about life at the home to determine whether the home meets the standards of practice as defined by OBRA.

The home receives a survey report explaining which aspects of the home are in compliance with the law, and which are not. This report is available in the nursing home so any visitor can review it. Sections of the survey report and information comparing facilities are available on the Internet at http://www.medicare.gov/Nursing/Overview.asp.

If a home doesn't follow the good standards of practice, it can be directed to make corrections immediately. The government can also issue fines, stop admissions until problems are corrected, regularly monitor the home to see that the corrections are made, or close the home.

But even with all these enforcement tools at its disposal, the government's ability to hold nursing homes to a good standard of care remains limited. Surveyors cannot be at the home all the time. They see only a snapshot of daily life when they are there.

What's more, budgetary constraints may make it less likely that government agencies will be able to visit as often and regulate as actively as they have in the past. Indeed, the law itself sometimes comes under attack in the Congress.

And that's where consumer advocates come in. Ombudsmen and families advocating for good care can be just as important in supporting good care as the government's regulatory role. As family members press the standards in the law in discussing care needs and approaches with nursing home staff, the law serves its intended purpose — as a tool for improvement in conditions.

You Are the Link to Better Care

Your first step toward good advocacy is to *continue to relate to your family member as you always have*. Nursing home residents often lose a sense of who they are because no one knows them. You're the link to the past, to your relative's identity. You can reinforce your relative's identity in your interactions with your relative and with staff.

Your second step is to *trust and act on your instincts*. Nursing home care is about taking care of human beings, people who have lived long, full lives and now need help in their last years. Because you know your relative, your insights are as important as the staff's skills. Together, you can help provide the care your relative needs.

It's natural to feel that if you bring concerns to the nursing home staff you will "rock the boat." Perhaps you might think: "This is what nursing homes are like." You might hesitate to speak up because your dad "has to live with the staff after I leave." Yet there are ways of bringing concerns to the staff that can make a big difference. This can be done without putting your parent at risk.

Many nursing home staff will welcome your constructive input. Remember that silence only allows problems to continue. If staff don't know your concerns, how can they address them? Chapter 7 offers guidance on bringing your concerns to the staff.

Third, *know your rights*. Then, you can act. It isn't easy. The perception among many people is that the nursing home knows how to take care of your Mom or Dad. If you determine that the facility isn't living up to your expectations, know that you have a right to voice your grievances, you and your relative have a right to participate in making decisions about care and daily life, and that you have a right to get help from the ombudsman program if you can't work things out directly with the nursing home.*

Fourth, take comfort in the fact that *laws, regulations and professional standards of good nursing home practice are on your side.* They provide clear requirements for nursing homes to respect residents' dignity and to provide compassionate, individualized care.

Finally, know that the laws work and care is better because of it. Nursing homes have improved their care over time. Through careful assessment, they're identifying each residents' strengths and frailties. They're designing plans of care that support a resident's ability to function. And everyone — staff, residents and families — sees the positive results.

☞ TIPS to Remember

1. Residents in today's nursing home have the same needs you would if you were living in a nursing home — a need for recognition as an individual — a very special individual human being.

2. Without this recognition, residents can feel homeless. This contributes to depression and withdrawal.

3. The best remedy is individualized care where staff get to know each resident and make adjustments in *facility* routines to support life-long *individual* routines.

4. Individualized care is the basic tenet of the standards established by the federal Nursing Home Reform law, and it applies to all nursing homes receiving federal money. It is the new standard of care.

5. Nursing home staff can provide individualized care by assessing each resident and developing a plan of care to meet that person's needs.

6. You can play a role by:

   • Sharing your knowledge of your relative with the nursing home staff; (In Appendix 5 you'll find a list of suggested information to share with staff to help them know your relative.)

---

*Contact The National Citizens' Coalition for Nursing Home Reform (see Appendix 7) for address of local/state advocacy group in your area.

- Participating in care planning meetings; and
- Expecting the home to make reasonable accommodations for your relative's individual needs and preferences.

7. Nursing homes need to be well-staffed to provide good care. And government agencies need sufficient resources to enforce the standards of care.

— All laws are subject to change. Regardless of any changes in the federal law discussed in this chapter, these standards are supported in some state laws as well as professional codes of conduct. They are good practice! They represent good care! As a family member you have every right to ask for and expect these practices for your relative. —

Anna's Story

ANNA HAD BEEN SYLVIA'S BEST FRIEND FROM THE AGE OF TEN. *Although Anna moved to the suburbs forty years ago, they'd still talked a couple times a week by phone. Even though Anna didn't live there anymore, she often knew the home town gossip days before her friend did.*

Anna had a series of strokes, each leaving her more paralyzed. Her husband Frank transformed their home into an accessible mini-hospital. Although Anna was depressed by her condition, she would be all made up, her hair just so, ready to play the hostess role for Sylvia's visits. The loss of the use of her right arm and leg didn't stop Anna from talking on the phone, continuing to insist on calling Sylvia back before she would talk with her.

Frank's third hernia operation meant he needed a six-week convalescence. The home health aide quit, unable to handle total care for Anna without Frank's help. Without other options, Frank arranged for Anna to be admitted to a nearby nursing home with a good reputation. He took her there the next day.

Sylvia visited the nursing home the following weekend, braced for the worst. When she'd spoken to Anna before she moved, Anna made it clear she didn't want to go. When Sylvia called her at the nursing home, the staff said she couldn't come to the phone.

Walking in the front door, Sylvia found a crowd of people in wheelchairs, some staring blankly into space, others slumped in their chairs. All seemed to be waiting, but for what it wasn't clear. Not finding Anna, Sylvia looked for a staff person to direct her to Anna's room. A woman touched her arm as Sylvia walked past. Sylvia turned and looked. "Anna?" she asked in disbelief. Anna's hair was combed, but had none of the usual flair. Her face was pale, peaked without her makeup. Awkwardly positioned, Anna was unable to adjust herself to look straight at Sylvia, so she tilted her head... and burst into tears.

Sylvia hugged and soothed her friend, and asked about a place to talk. Anna was too worried about her husband Frank. "I haven't heard from him all day. Where is he? I know something's wrong. I just know he's lying on the floor.

"I'll call him for you," Sylvia said. "And I'll find out what's going on. But first let us take you some place where we can talk."

As they moved toward Anna's room, Sylvia introduced herself to an aide and asked where she and Anna could talk in private. One of the aides pointed to a room down the hall. After Sylvia found the pay phone and learned that Frank was okay, she reported back to Anna.

The two friends talked for awhile. About 4:30, Anna had to go to the bathroom. It took half an hour to get assistance because the staff members were rushing around with the medications and the trays for the evening meal. Eventually, someone helped her and then they were able to go to the dining room for dinner.

Anna said she didn't have an appetite, that she hadn't eaten since she'd arrived. After reminding Anna to eat to keep up her strength, she realized that the real problem wasn't one of the will, but of the way. This night's main course was pasta twirls, a challenge for the most able-bodied eaters, but a frustrating embarrassment for a naturally right-handed person now forced to eat with her left hand. As food landed in her lap, Anna apologized for her mess. The one aide in the room appeared overwhelmed assisting people to and from their tables. Most of those in the dining room had no one to help them eat.

Sylvia coaxed and fed her friend, helping her to get most of the meal down. Anna wouldn't drink the whole milk offered; she was used to low-fat milk. Anna lamented that she was supposed to be on a low-cholesterol, low-fat diet, but the home's physician had issued orders for a regular diet.

Anna's table mate was cheerful and warm, and with Sylvia's prompting, they struck up a conversation. As they left the dining room, Sylvia sought some reassurance that the woman would eat with Anna again, and then took her friend back to her room. "Please, get me out of here," Anna pleaded, amid tears, hugs, apologies and thanks.

On subsequent visits, Sylvia found that the situation didn't improve for Anna. Anna withdrew, grew weaker, and lost her spirit.

In lots of little ways, this "good" nursing home contributed to Anna's deterioration. But it didn't have to be that way.

If Sylvia had known how to advocate for her friend, she could have helped bring concerns to the attention of the staff. With proper assessment and care planning, the situation could have improved. Staff would have known enough about Anna to individualize her care and her routines. If this nursing home had been following the standards in the law, things would have been different. Staff would've known:

• *Anna's connection to the outside world, via the telephone, was critical to her morale. Therefore, extra efforts would have been made to get phone calls through to her and assist her in making calls. Staff would have talked with Anna about the possibility of having a phone by her bedside, as she'd had in her own home.*

• *Anna's spirits were always directly linked to her appearance. Staff would've helped her maintain her hairstyle and makeup, as a basic part of her grooming. They would know these were essential to her well-being.*

• *Anna required assistance to eat and a diet suited to her individual nutritional needs and restrictions. She needed meals to accommodate her limited left-handed abilities, occupational therapy to increase the agility of her left hand, and silverware suitable for her unsteady grip.*

• *Anna thrived on social contact and needed help making friends. If she could have been actively engaged in meaningful relationships she would have managed to feel less lonely and isolated, more comfortable and at home.*

Chapter 2

Cornerstone of Care:
Residents' Rights

- **Step Up** — Know your rights.
  - **Speak Up** — Residents must be treated with dignity.
    - **Advocate for Good Care** — Participate in care planning.

"I just got sick of the way the staff was ignoring me and always turning to my son for decisions as if I were incompetent. Finally, my son had to tell them to ask me."
— nursing home resident, Denver CO

WHAT IS IT THAT PEOPLE FEAR MOST ABOUT NURSING homes? *The prospect of having to yield their freedom, privacy, choice, independence and control.*

It's the "little" things — savoring an early morning cup of coffee, meeting a friend for lunch, watching a late movie — that people miss the most if these are no longer possible. Living in a nursing home can completely disrupt lifelong routines, and greatly diminish options for personal choice. Because of these factors, residents need support and encouragement to exercise their rights to make as many decisions about their daily lives as possible.

And that's where you come in.

Why are There Residents' Rights?

Federal nursing home law and many state laws contain specific provisions that protect residents' rights — the basic human and civil liberties that most of us take for granted every day. For example: the right to visit with anyone you choose, or the right to get up and go to bed when you wish. Who wouldn't expect to make such decisions? You don't lose any rights when you move into a nursing home.

But nursing home staff tend to focus on routine and efficiency. They must care for large numbers of frail, dependent people. Respect for the rights of individual residents sometimes gets lost in the drive to operate efficiently as a business.

The nursing home is an institution, with institutional bureaucracy and management. Staff may be hurried, have too many residents to care for, residents are physically frail and often mentally confused. These factors help explain why the law places so much emphasis on residents' rights.

Residents' rights are one of the key items state survey agencies must inspect during their reviews of nursing homes. Many have their own strict laws and regulations to protect individual rights. (You can learn more about the survey process in chapter 7, "Problem Solving: Being Your Own Advocate.")

Residents and their families generally receive a copy of a home's policy on residents' rights upon admission. This important document can help residents receive the best possible care. It's a good idea for both residents and family members to reread it from time to time. A summary of federal residents' rights appears in Appendix 3. Be sure the home's policy does not violate rights you are entitled to.

☞   TIP — If you don't have a copy of the residents' rights, by all means ask for it! Homes also prominently post it.

Let's take a look at some of the major rights guaranteed to residents of nursing homes.

Whose Rights?

Our emphasis here, of course, is on the rights of *residents*. Staff, families and physicians have rights, too, and all have important roles to play. But when a person moves into a nursing home, it's common for everyone *but* the resident to assume a decision-making role. That's unfortunate, because the quickest way to send someone into depression is to seize her right to make choices about the course of her own life. Your role as a family member is to assist your relative in exercising her rights. You fulfill your role best when you look at life from your relative's perspective.

> — The quickest way to send someone into depression is to seize her right to make choices about the course of her own life. —

Sadly, many residents are denied their rights by their own inability to make decisions. Experts estimate that 60-80% of the people living in nursing homes today have some degree of mental impairment. Still, even people who are forgetful or confused can express their needs and wants. Often a resident who needs help with complex matters may be able to make her own decisions about day-to-day issues. The resident's ability to communicate may be better on some days than on others, but such fluctuations shouldn't interfere with the basic right to express feelings and exercise choice to the greatest degree possible.

Residents Who Can't Choose

Residents who are completely unable to participate effectively in their own care need to have a substitute decision-maker, or advocate, to ensure their rights are protected. A close family member is usually in the best position to understand — and to help staff understand — what the resident might say or choose if she were able to express her own preferences. What, for example, is her usual morning routine? What does she normally eat for breakfast? What kind of music does she enjoy?

What are the Rights of Residents?

Under federal standards, residents' rights include the right to:
- receive information
- participate in planning all aspects of care
- make choices and independent personal decisions
- enjoy privacy in care and confidentiality regarding medical, personal or financial affairs
- be treated with dignity and respect
- know personal possessions are safe and secure
- be protected against transfer, unless for specific reasons
- raise concerns or complaints.

Knowing the rights is an important first step, but it's not enough. What's really important is *exercising* these rights. Chapter 7's discussion on problem solving describes the steps to take when a resident or advocate thinks the resident's rights have been violated. That chapter offers information about how, when, and where to call for help and guidance in getting the problem resolved.

In this chapter, the focus is on the rights themselves and what they mean to residents in nursing homes.

The Right to Information

Besides giving residents a copy of their rights on admission to the nursing home, the facility must provide other kinds of information, including material that explains:
- services available in the facility
- state laws regarding living wills, durable powers of attorney for health care and other forms of advance directives, along with the facility's policy on carrying out these directives
- *all* matters related to financial charges, including a list specifically indicating what items are covered by Medicaid or by the daily private-pay rate
- the Medicaid application process
- the amount of money a Medicaid resident has in his/her personal needs account (residents should regularly receive statements with this information)
- how to review the most recent survey of the facility by the licensure or certification agency
- how to examine a resident's medical records (a resident may transfer this authority to another person either through consent or through legal authority).

In addition, the facility also should provide information, including addresses and telephone numbers, on how to reach:
- the state licensure and certification agency
- the local and state long-term care ombudsman
- the area's protection and advocacy organization (the agencies that investigate abuse).

During admission, residents and their families typically receive an enormous amount of new information. You'll want to be able to easily find this information if needed.

☞ TIP — It's a good idea for friends and families to set up a small filing system to keep track of these important papers and bills.

Here's an example of the right to information regarding charges.

Your mother is on Medicaid. At the end of the first month of her stay in the nursing home, you receive a bill for adult incontinence briefs. Is this cost covered by Medicaid in your state?

Under federal law, the nursing home must provide you information on covered costs. If you pay privately, the facility must inform you of all charges for any services not included in the daily rate.

The Right to Participate in Planning and Care

All nursing home residents are entitled to take part in planning for their own care. (A detailed explanation of the care planning process appears in chapter 3.) Residents have the following rights of participation in this important process:

- to be fully informed, in advance, and participate in making decisions about all care and treatment and any changes in that care and treatment that may affect residents' well-being
- to participate in their own care planning meetings
- to refuse treatment and to receive information regarding appropriate alternatives
- to self-administer medication, if the interdisciplinary assessment team determines this is safe
- to privacy and confidentiality with regard to medical records
- to be free from vest restraints, hand mitts, seat belts and other physical restraints
- to be free from unnecessary antipsychotic drugs, sedatives and other chemical restraints.

Looking at this list you can see the importance of talking with facility staff from the very beginning about your relative's wants and needs. You and your relative need to be involved in assessing needs, setting goals and planning for care. In chapter 3 you'll learn why a care planning meeting is a good time to discuss the issues listed above.

— Nursing home residents are the best judges of their own bodies. —

Understanding and being vocal in this process are keys to ensuring good care. You can also ask for a family meeting with staff in between care planning meetings.

Generally, nursing home residents are the best judges of their own bodies. Unless severely impaired, residents know when they are thirsty, hungry, or need to go to the bathroom. They know when they don't feel right because of a certain medicine. They know that appropriate movement and exercise, adjusted for ability, builds strength, confidence and a sense of well-being.

Sometimes it's necessary to remind staff caregivers that residents should be in charge of their own bodies. Residents usually can tell the staff caregivers when, and how, to help.

Your father is in the nursing home to recover from a stroke. He tells you that the new medication his doctor has prescribed makes him very dizzy. When he refused to take it yesterday, the nurse became angry and practically forced it in his mouth.

Your father has the right to question the effects of medication and to refuse to take it. This is the time to speak to the nurse or to the doctor on your father's behalf.

The Right to Make Independent Choices

Studies show that one of the most important factors in nursing facility residents' quality of life is the ability to continue to make choices about their own lives. Living in a nursing home does not take away a person's right to an individual schedule. Some activities may be modified but shouldn't jeopardize respect for a resident's preferences. Although the following list isn't spelled out in the law, the right to choice clearly includes:

- getting up and going to bed when a resident chooses
- eating or enjoying a variety of snacks outside of regularly scheduled meal times (within dietary restrictions)
- selecting what to wear
- choosing activities, deciding how to spend time, and receiving a choice in main meals
- managing personal finances (when possible).

— Residents should be taken — or able to go — to the bathroom when they need to go, not just when the time is convenient for staff. —

Some people have eaten large breakfasts throughout their lives, while others may simply like a cup of coffee, juice and toast in the morning. Some are early risers, others prefer to sleep later. Residents should be able to choose their morning fare and when to wake up and go to bed.

The federal law directs facilities to provide residents "reasonable accommodation of needs." Of course, this mandate does not mean repainting walls to satisfy residents' and families' decorating tastes. But the law does require that the home's activities should meet a variety of interests. It means that food should be prepared to meet individual tastes and needs. Sleep should be interrupted only for necessary care. Residents should be taken — or able to go — to the bathroom when they need to go, not just when the time is convenient for staff.

> *Whenever you visit your mother in the morning, you notice she can hardly stay awake. She says that staff wake her up so early that by 10 a.m. she's worn out. You discover that the nurse assistants on the night shift get her up at 5 a.m. to get dressed. Then she waits in the hall in her wheelchair until breakfast at 8 o'clock!*
>
> *When you inquire about this situation, you're told that "the day shift doesn't have time to get everyone up."*
>
> *Staff are out of line here, and should be instructed that your mother has the right to get up according to her own wishes.*

The Right to Privacy

The loss of privacy is one of the main fears among people who face living in a nursing home. Moving into a nursing home usually means sharing a room with a stranger. The residents are expected to get along despite differences in their conditions, personalities and, perhaps, culture. The space allocated to each resident is often barely large enough for a bed, small table, and chair. Although curtains may be drawn between the beds, they don't shut out sounds, making private conversations difficult.

Privacy is often lost amid the brisk pace and commotion of the caregiving routine. Staff may enter a room without knocking or waiting for a response to the knock. They might take a resident down the hall to the bath without making sure that the person is fully clothed.

Good care, however, demands a different scene, granting residents specific privacy rights, including the right to privacy in:

- treatment
- caring for personal needs
- visits with family and friends
- communication — such as when making or receiving telephone calls and sending or receiving mail unopened

- personal matters, such as medical condition and financial affairs.

These required accommodations to residents' basic privacy needs thus provide that there must be a place to make a phone call without being disturbed or overheard, and a quiet place to visit with friends and family. Staff must make sure that doors are closed and curtains pulled during care treatments, and that residents aren't exposed when their roommate has visitors or when they're sitting in the hall or going to the bath. Residents' mail must not be opened without their consent.

> When you are visiting your mother in the nursing home, staff members often enter the room and interrupt your privacy. Your mother also tells you that someone is always walking in, even when the door is closed, just when she is dressing or going to the bathroom.
>
> You should bring these problems to staff's attention and remind them that residents are entitled to a knock and an affirmative response before staff members enter the room.

The Right to Dignity

Nursing home residents rank the way staff treat them as the most important factor in their care. Nothing is more valuable to residents than staff who are kind, courteous and respectful. Residents want a well-trained staff whom they can know and trust. They want to receive help when they need it. They want to be spoken to like adults. They want to be treated with dignity.

— *Nursing home residents rank the way staff treat them as the most important factor in their care.* —

> Your mother tells you that the aide on the 3 to 11 p.m. shift is mean to her. She tells your mother to shut up, and that she doesn't have time to take her to the bathroom again.
>
> You know that the standard of care is that facilities support each resident's quality of life. You also know that the facility must provide care in a way that maintains or enhances each resident's dignity.
>
> You should inform administration about the problem with the aide and ask for their commitment to deal with the situation.

The Right to Freedom of Association

The constitutional right to speak to and associate with whomever one chooses doesn't vanish when one moves into a nursing home. But, sometimes, well-meaning family and staff attempt to interfere with a resident's relationships. Residents have the right to:

- share a room with a spouse
- gather with other residents and resident groups within the home without staff being present
- meet with state and local ombudsmen or any agency providing advocacy or services
- belong to any church or social group
- receive visitors at reasonable hours
- leave the nursing home
- make or receive telephone calls.

An old friend of your mother comes in to visit her at the nursing home at least once a week. The staff tell you that after every visit your mother seems to be very upset. They think that the friend tells your mother that she doesn't need to be in the nursing home.

The issue here is whether your mother wants to see her friend. If she does, she has the right to see her, whether she is upset or not. Neither the nursing home nor you retains the right to limit visitors.

Rights Regarding Transfer and Discharge

Few aspects of nursing home care can be more traumatic than when a resident is told to leave the home or move to another room. With good reason, families and residents dread these two situations. To have to adjust to a different facility or even to a different room and roommate usually is disruptive and distressful for everyone.

Facilities are required to follow specific procedures for transfers and discharges. You can minimize the distress of a transfer by making yourself aware of the rights of residents — and the policies of the facility which should reflect the law — regarding transfer and discharge.

Reasons for Transfer or Discharge. Transfers are permissible only under certain reasons and conditions. These include:

- when the resident's health or safety is endangered in the facility

- when, after reasonable notice, a bill for care remains unpaid
- when it is necessary for the resident's welfare because the resident's needs cannot be met in the nursing home
- when it is appropriate because the resident's health has improved enough that the resident no longer needs the facility's services.

Notification. Before a resident can be transferred, the facility must notify the resident, family member or legal representative in writing. The facility must give the *reasons for the move* and *30 days' notice*, except in certain emergencies. The notice must include:

- a statement indicating that the resident has a right to appeal this action
- the name, address and telephone number of the state long-term care ombudsman.

(A note to residents of sub-acute/short term units: Even if you signed admission papers agreeing to transfer when your Medicare coverage runs out, you are entitled to contest the transfer at a hearing. Talk to your ombudsman for assistance.)

The facility must assist the resident to prepare for the move and provide whatever services are necessary to protect the resident's safety and arrange for an appropriate plan after discharge.

Room-to-room transfer. A facility may ask an individual to change rooms for a variety of reasons: to resolve roommate issues, to accommodate a new resident, because of a change in the resident's level of care or source of payment.

Even a transfer to a nearby room can be exceedingly difficult when a resident has become familiar with her particular space and place. Typically, a resident doesn't have the same right of appeal as in the case of a transfer out of the facility.

— *If the purpose of a move is to relocate within a Medicare wing or from a Medicare wing, a resident may refuse to transfer.* —

However, the facility must accommodate the needs of each particular resident and residents have the right to make choices about aspects of life that are important to them. By moving a resident from one room to another, the facility may be failing to meet these requirements. If the purpose of a move is to relocate within a Medicare wing or from a Medicare wing, a resident may refuse to transfer and may be entitled to a hearing.

Transfer to hospital. When a resident is transferred to a hospital, the home must give the resident and family a written notice explaining its policy on holding beds. The policy should say how long the bed will be held and how much will be charged to hold it. Facilities must readmit residents participating in Medicaid to the first available semi-private room.

> *Marla's father has Alzheimer's disease, and has been living at Sunset Care for three months. He had a rough time adjusting at first, but has accepted his new surroundings and resolved to make the best of them. Marla has noticed, however, that he has grown increasingly agitated in the last few weeks.*
>
> *Now the Director of Nurses is on the phone to Marla, telling her that Sunset Care cannot continue to care for her father, and asking that she find a new facility for him within three days! When Marla asks why, the director says her father is wandering into other people's rooms and threatening them. The message throws Marla into a panic. She is an only child and her father is a widower. Marla has a full-time job and two small children. What should she do? What are her rights? What are her father's rights?*
>
> *Sunset Care has failed to give the required thirty-days notice of discharge, and to inform Marla and her father of their right to appeal the transfer. Marla needs help from someone who knows the federal and state regulations on discharge. She can call the local or state ombudsman or seek guidance from the agency that licenses nursing homes. She can request a hearing to contest the transfer. Often, a conference or outside consultation can encourage the nursing home to reexamine its decision and find out the reason Marla's father is entering other resident's rooms.(See chapter 5 for discussion on wandering.)*

☞ TIP — Find out how to contact your local and state Long-Term Care Ombudsman Programs and State Licensing Agencies *before you need them.* Contact information is in Appendix 7.

The Right to Security for Possessions

With the many losses residents endure when entering a nursing home, it would be ideal if they could have familiar room furnishings around them. Residents do have the right to bring their own things into the nursing home, as space permits. The problem, of course, is that there usually isn't much space. Personal possessions, alas, are frequently misplaced or stolen. Consequently, nursing homes advise people to leave anything of value behind with relatives or to store small items, such as jewelry, in a safe in the facility. Some nursing homes have locked drawers or cabinets in residents' rooms. Other homes are willing to remove the institutional furniture and encourage residents bring their own.

One of the most common complaints from residents and families relates to lost clothing. Was it lost in the laundry or taken by mistake? Did it simply disappear mysteriously? Missing articles don't have to be an accepted feature of nursing home life. Many nursing homes pay serious attention to reports of missing items and have specific follow-up procedures.

Those facilities with fewer cases of lost property usually have the same staff permanently assigned to the same residents. They become protective of resident's personal belongings. These facilities also involve staff in working toward residents' care goals.

☞ TIP — Take an inventory upon admission. Residents and families should keep a copy. Clothes and dentures should be appropriately marked for identification. Update the list when changes are made.

If a possession is missing:
• give the facility a written request for locating the missing possession and include an expected date for a reply;
• ask what the home's policy is for replacement of lost articles. Some homes have insurance policies to cover larger items.

☞ TIP — You may wish to extend your homeowner's insurance policy to the resident's belongings.

Your grandmother has been in Rosehips Care Center for two months. Over that period of time, two dresses, her afghan and four pairs of hosiery have been lost. When you ask staff about it, they say you must accept that these things happen in a nursing home.

The fact is that you need not accept such a situation. You should expect that staff will take responsibility for locating or replacing lost items. It would be helpful to discuss this problem in a resident or family council meeting, or both.

Keep in mind that a nursing home is part of the community and problems involving stolen items may need to involve the local police.

The Right to Raise Concerns

The problems that arise in nursing homes are frequent, varied and complex. Most concern basic care, and often stem from staffing. Short staffing and high turnover rates may result in call lights left unanswered, residents bathed sporadically, and staff too busy to help residents with meals.

— Keep in mind that a nursing home is part of the community and problems involving stolen items may need to involve the local police. —

Staff attitude and behavior toward residents are common sources of resident complaints. Hurried grooming services or care treatments and thoughtless or abusive staff language affect the dignity and self-worth of residents. You wouldn't put up with it from your barber or your next-door neighbor; why should that change when you move into a nursing home?

Many times staff do not realize that the language they are accustomed to using at home, that they may have grown up with, that they use with their children, sounds harsh and frightening to an older person who never used "shut up." This language is not acceptable and can be considered verbal abuse. It points out the need for staff education and training.

Verbal as well as physical abuse should be reported to the administration. Most facilities will take immediate steps to investigate and correct the situation.

Fear of Complaining

It is important to recognize and appreciate a resident's fear of retaliation. An individual who lives twenty-four hours a day totally dependent on caregivers may feel that challenging or offending those caregivers, or making repeated requests, may make them even less

— It is important to recognize and appreciate a resident's fear of retaliation. —

likely to respond to his needs. As one family member remarked: "I felt the same way when my children were in school. I was afraid to complain to the teacher for fear he would take it out on my son."

It's true there are instances where residents suffer indignities because they or their families have expressed their concerns. Indeed, they may be labeled as "chronic complainers." After all, staff may find it easier to label someone than to take the time to address that person's special needs.

But fear of complaining is often unjustified. Indeed, raising concerns is essential to receiving better care. Residents, family members and ombudsmen agree that being assertive and identifying problems usually brings good results. Becoming directly involved in care planning, as discussed in chapter 3, is one of the best ways for you and your relative to ensure rights are respected.

☞ TIP — It's not what you say, it's how you say it! Expressing your concerns in a friendly-but-firm assertive manner will usually be much more effective than making aggressive demands.

Facility Responsibility

Every nursing home has a responsibility to make sure that residents and staff are aware of residents' rights. This entails assisting residents in raising concerns individually, in resident councils, or in care planning meetings. The facility is required to respond promptly to these concerns.

> *When Betty visits her mother, she often finds her sitting in urine or stool. Betty has taken her concerns to the aides and the charge nurses who frequently tell her that they just don't have enough staff that day. She also has gone to the administrator several times. On the last occasion, Betty was told that, if she is dissatisfied, she "may wish to find another nursing home."*
>
> *This response signifies the facility's unwillingness to address the problem. It may be time to call for outside help. Chapter 7 offers specific ideas and resources for solving such problems.*

Step Up, Speak Up, and Advocate for Good Care
- Know that *privacy* means that curtains must be drawn when care is given!
- Know that *participation in care planning* means a serious consideration of resident views and concerns!
- Know that *being treated with dignity* means being taken seriously and not being labeled a "complainer!"
- Know that *your relative's rights regarding transfers* mean that she can't be asked to leave because you or she raised concerns!

- Know that *your relative's right to choices* means that she can decide whether to play Bingo or take a nap!

This chapter has touched on just a few key aspects of nursing home residents' rights and how to seek help in exercising those rights. Residents' rights is a theme that steers virtually every aspect of nursing home care, from admission to discharge. The

> — *The most critical thing to remember is that residents retain their basic right to be in control of their lives.* —

most critical thing to remember is that *residents retain their basic right to be in control of their lives.* Living in a nursing home does not take away that right!

In the next chapter, "Assessment and Care Planning: Receiving Individualized Care," you will learn more specifics about how you and your relative can have an active role in planning care and treatment. Assessment and care planning are concrete ways a resident can exercise the right to participation and maintain some choice and control. Read on for lots of ideas about making rights a daily reality!

> — *All laws are subject to change. Regardless of any changes in the federal law discussed in this chapter, these standards are supported in some state laws as well as professional codes of conduct. They are good practice! They represent good care! As a family member you have every right to ask for and expect these practices for your relative.* —

Chapter 3

Assessment and Care Planning: Receiving Individualized Care

- **Step Up** — and join in planning care.
  - **Speak Up** — and individualize care.
    - **Advocate for Good Care** — and monitor the implementation.

Whenever you visit your mother, Mrs. Bailey, she says she misses her daily walk outside. She also says she has trouble going to sleep without her nightly bath, a routine she found so relaxing. Because she frequently mentions these feelings, you know these two lifelong patterns are important. You wish there were something you could do.

THERE IS SOMETHING YOU CAN DO! YOUR MOTHER'S CONCERNS can be addressed in her *care plan*. This plan for her care and treatment is based on an assessment conducted by the nursing facility staff. Later in this chapter you'll see how your mother's lifelong patterns fit into her care plan. First, however, an explanation of care planning and assessment will help you know what you need to do. Think of these as *keys* for getting individualized care for your mother.

What Are the Keys?
Assessment and care planning are the keys to good care. The assessment process is the key to information about what each individual needs to maintain physical, mental, and social function. Care planning is the key to addressing those needs identified during the assessment. Both the assessment process and care planning were established in the federal law as standards of good nursing home practice to achieve each residents' right to individualized care.

The preceding chapter on residents' rights discussed the right to participate in planning care and the importance of talking with staff. Assessment and care planning are two excellent opportunities for resident and family participation! They provide a time for discussion and asking questions.

What Is the Assessment Process?

An assessment process is a way to collect factual information about an individual. Assessments are conducted by nursing home staff with information from the resident's physician and other specialists. Typically, an assessment includes staff from these departments: nursing, social services, activities, dietary and sometimes the therapies. Participation from residents and family members is essential to this process. The assessment process will probably occur over a period of days, with staff members making observations and talking with both the resident and family.

During an assessment information is gathered about various aspects of an individual's life and abilities.

An assessment determines an individual's:

- **abilities** in areas such as:

walking	talking	eating	dressing
bathing	seeing	hearing	understanding
remembering			

- **assistance needs:** how much assistance, if any, is needed in each area
- **patterns and preferences** in areas such as:

daily routines	activities	habits	relationships

Once this basic information is collected, staff ask why limitations in function exist. What is causing the limitation?

While assessing your mother, a nurse asks her to walk across the room. Mrs. Bailey takes slow, cautious steps. She reaches out to steady herself. The nurse knows unsteadiness could be caused by various factors including medications, constant sitting, weak muscles, shoes that don't fit, a urinary infection, or even an earache. To help your mother improve her ability to walk, the nurse must determine the specific cause of your mother's unsteadiness. Your mother's doctor, a physical therapist, nurse assistants, and others might be needed to help identify the cause of the unsteadiness.

When Are Assessments Conducted?

Good professional practice and the law require:

- **an assessment** usually within **fourteen days** of admission*

---

* In a Medicare skilled nursing unit the initial assessment is completed within 5 days of admission.

- **a reassessment** whenever there is a **significant change** in the resident's condition, either an improvement or decline
- **a review** of some sections of the assessment every **three months** (quarterly)
- **an annual reassessment** completed within twelve months of the most recent full assessment.

What Is a Resident's Role in the Assessment Process?

Residents need to help staff get to know them. Residents should tell staff their needs and hopes and how they feel. A complete assessment process for Mrs. Bailey would include information about the following areas.

Strengths (physical, social, spiritual): What does she have to build upon? What does she do well? How does she solve problems and overcome hardships? What talents and skills does she have? Does she find strength in her faith?

Daily, customary routines: When does she usually awaken? When does she go to sleep? Does she awaken during the night to go to the bathroom? Does she prefer showers or baths? Does she go out every week? Does she have a pet? What is a typical day like for her? What are things that will make each day a good day?

- **Preferences:** What is important to her regarding her activities? Care? Food?
- **Abilities:** What is her ability to stand, to walk, to dress herself?
- **Feedback:** What is her relationship with her roommate? Do they get along? How are things going in her relationships with family and friends? Honest answers are necessary for staff to understand how to work with her.

What As the Family's Role in the Assessment Process?

As a family member or close friend of a resident, staff may ask you for information about the resident's abilities, needs, habits, and relationships. Of course, your relative's permission is needed for you to talk with the staff about her. Appendix 4, "I Want to Tell You About My Mother," illustrates the type of information you might offer that could be very helpful to the staff and your relative. The more information that the resident and family members share with staff, the better prepared they'll be to give good care.

Within two weeks of Mrs. Bailey entering the nursing home, staff should have learned a great deal about her by observing and by talking with both of you. Through the assessment process, they would have learned that Mrs. Bailey likes to walk outside every day and take baths at night. They would use this information when planning care with your mother.

Care Planning

Once the assessment process lays a foundation of facts, staff construct ways to meet an individual's needs. *Care planning* is the process of building *a plan of care to meet needs.*

What Is a Plan of Care?

A plan of care is the strategy for how the staff will help a resident. It says what each staff person will do and when it will happen. To picture how this works, think back to the opening scenario.

To address your mother's concerns, her care plan might include the following statements: "The nurse assistant on the afternoon shift will help Mrs. Bailey outside for a fifteen-minute walk each day. Mrs. Bailey will be assisted to a bath instead of a shower, every evening at 8 p.m., by the nurse assistant assigned to her care.

For a care plan to succeed, a resident must think the plan meets her needs and must be comfortable with it. A care plan can address any medical or non-medical problem such as incompatibility with a roommate, as illustrated here:

Your dad is distressed because his roommate talks non-stop. Your dad needs more quiet. The care plan goal for this need might be to find a compatible roommate. In the interim, staff could help your dad find a place where he can be alone during part of the day. Another action step on the plan might be getting your dad a radio/cassette player with earphones. A third action could involve having the activities professional encourage your dad's roommate to participate in a discussion group with other residents. The introduction of this activity could change the care plan for your dad's roommate and lead to other ways to accommodate his need to talk.

What's In a Care Plan?

All care plans have the same basic information. They should be written using words that everyone can understand. When you look at a care plan, you should be able to know:

- the individual's problems or needs: What does the resident need?
- the goal for each problem or need: What are the resident and staff working to achieve? What's the result?
- the approaches to be used to reach each goal: *What* is to be done? *When* will it be done? *How* will the goal be met? *Who* will do it?
- the timetable for meeting or reevaluating the goal: When will the need be met? When will this approach be evaluated to see if it's working? Is the goal realistic?
- the staff person with the key responsibility for each approach to whom you should go if some adjustments need to be made: Who will help the resident? Who is responsible for overseeing each goal? (See "Who's Who in the Staff" on page 4.)

☞ TIP—Many care plans are generated by computers which list the resident's *problems* and suggestions for generic approaches and goals that do not reflect the person. If you discuss the resident's *needs* and approaches that build on the resident's patterns and preferences, you will help staff *individualize* care for your loved one.

How Can You Tell a Good Care Plan from a Bad One?

A good care plan will:
- be specific, individualized, and written in common language everyone can understand

- reflect the resident's concerns and preference and support the resident's well-being, functioning and rights

A bad care plan will:
- be written in medical terms with general goals and approaches that don't reflect the residents' preferences and individuality

- ignore the resident's ideas or wishes, label the resident's choices or needs as *problems* or *problem behaviors*

- use an interdisciplinary team approach and tap resources outside the facility as needed

- be written by one staff person with other staff agreeing; no "give and take" among staff about needs and approaches

- change as the resident's needs change

- stay the same, with no changes in goals or approaches

How Are Care Plans Developed?

Care plans are developed and reviewed through a process of discussion, usually in meetings called *care planning conferences.* This meeting is a time for staff, residents, family members or resident representatives to have a dialogue. It is a time to being up problems, ask questions, and offer information to help staff provide care to meet the resident's needs. Residents and their family or legal representatives must be invited to attend their care planning meeting.

Successful care planning involves many people, including:

- the resident
- family member(s), friends, advocates, or any other people the resident requests
- an interdisciplinary treatment team, which includes the resident's personal physician, nurse, social worker, nurse assistants, pharmacist, therapists, and others as needed
- all nursing home staff who provide direct care to the resident.

Any of these key participants who are unable to be present at the care planning conference should submit written comments and ideas for the care plan.

☞ TIP—Nurse assistants are often very helpful in care planning meetings. They typically have a wealth of information about the resident and ideas about approaches that work.

When Are Care Planning Conferences Held?

- *Following an assessment:* A care plan must be developed or reviewed within seven days after a new assessment is completed.

• *Quarterly:* A care plan review for each resident should occur every three months to see if the plan is working and if any changes need to be made in it.

• *As needed:* A care plan needs to be reviewed whenever there is a major change in a resident's physical or mental health that might require a change in care.

Consider, for example:

Your mother's roommate, Mrs. Cornelius, says that her doctor changed her medicine and told her she would be receiving some physical therapy. She doesn't think his orders are being followed, but doesn't want to bother the nurses with questions because they always are so busy.

When the doctor changed Mrs. Cornelius's medicine and ordered physical therapy for her, her care plan should have changed. Facility staff should discuss the changes with her so they can agree on a course of action. As the new medicine is given, staff should ask her questions to see how the medicine is working. If there are problems, staff should contact her doctor to see whether any changes are needed.

The resident or you can request a care plan conference whenever you think a review is needed. Going back to the original question posed in this chapter, as Mrs. Bailey's child, what can you do?

When your mother tells you about missing her daily walks outside and her evening baths, ask the supervising nurse for a care planning conference to discuss these issues with the staff. Together with the staff, your mother and you come up with some ways to continue her routines and agree on the one most acceptable to her. Your mother's care plan is changed to incorporate these routines. Care planning is an appropriate setting for this discussion because resuming these daily routines might involve staff from more than one department and might affect some other aspects of your mother's schedule.

How Can You Support a Resident in a Care Planning Meeting?

The Setting. As a family member of a nursing home resident, it is extremely important to help your relative participate in planning for care. A resident might need support from family members, friends, or an ombudsman to discuss needs, preferences, and wishes in care planning meetings. Sitting at a table with several professional staff members responsible for your care can be very intimidating. A resident has a right to choose someone to go with him to the care plan meeting.

Resident's Perspective. A resident who cannot, or does not choose to, participate in care planning, may appoint a representative — perhaps you. Facility staff need to hear how things are going from the *resident's* perspective. If there are questions, staff members need you to help answer them. If there are problems, staff need your ideas on how to solve them. It is desirable to involve the resident in care planning as much as possible, including residents with dementia. Always assume that the resident may understand aspects of the care planning conference and, on some level, be able to communicate any concerns.

Resident Focus. Remember that care planning is for the resident. The resident's opinions, desires, and decisions need to be heard and respected. What the resident wants may not always be what the staff recommends or what you as a family member would choose. As you either support or represent your relative in planning for care, *be sure that your relative's views are voiced and honored.* After all, it is the resident who lives in the facility twenty-four hours a day, seven days a week. Without the resident's agreement, it is more difficult, if not impossible, to achieve the goals of the care plan.

— Be sure that your relative's views are voiced and honored. —

Advance Planning. To help the resident's wants and needs be properly addressed, residents and families must plan ahead for the conference. Offer some assistance with this preparation by asking the resident to describe, or observe for yourself, a typical day in the nursing home. Does it build upon the *resident's* strengths, daily routines and preferences? If there are concerns or problems, how would *the resident* like them addressed? You can help your relative prepare by calling attention to the points listed in the next section, and to such everyday issues as air quality (smoke, smells), noise, privacy, toilet schedules, food service and quality, cleanliness, freedom of choice, staff attitude, or responsiveness to concerns.

How Can a Resident Participate in Care Planning?

Residents can and should take an active role in care planning. The points below provide guidance to enable residents and/or their advocates to prepare for and join in care planning. A section is also included telling what to do if there are problems in the follow through on the care plan.

Before the Meeting a Resident and/or Advocate Should
Be informed about needs, care and treatment.

Know or ask the primary care physician or nursing or other staff about his condition and treatment plan.

Ask questions if more information is needed **Review personal records** and ask for assistance in understanding the information if necessary.

Ask staff to hold the meeting when family members can come, if the resident wants you there.

Plan a personal agenda for the meeting. Make a list of questions to ask and note the help needed. Identify the important needs or concerns to discuss. Clarify goals. Share them with a key staff member.

During the Meeting a Resident and/or Advocate Can
Discuss options for treatment and for meeting his needs and preferences.

If necessary, **ask if there are other ways** to perform a procedure or meet a goal.

Suggest at least a couple of ways the resident's needs or wishes can be met. **Be open to trying new things,** at least on a short-term basis. **Ask staff to explore alternate ways** to accomplish the resident's goal if it is difficult to reach agreement.

Mr. Dupree says bathing in the whirlpool scares him. Is there another way to keep him clean and give good skin care? The care planning team suggested other possibilities and he chose the one he found most agreeable.

Ask for more information, or another explanation, to better understand what is proposed or why. You and the resident should have a clear grasp of the choices. **Ask questions** whenever an explanation of terms or procedures is needed. Remember: No question is too simple!

Understand and agree with the care plan before the meeting ends. If the resident disagrees with a problem the staff identifies, he should ask staff to show him how they have determined (assessed) the existing problem.

The resident may refuse the care plan goals that staff identify, or he may refuse some of staff's suggested approaches for meeting goals. Staff must talk with the resident about treatment decisions, such as medications. Staff can only do what the resident agrees is acceptable.

Consider these questions:
- Does the plan meet the resident's individual needs and goals?
- Is the resident willing to work toward accomplishing these goals?
- Are the approaches compatible with the resident's schedule and preferences?
- Does the plan give the resident enough information to know whether it is being followed?

Remember to ask for:
- a copy of the care plan.
- the name of the staff member to speak with if something on the care plan needs to be changed.

After the Meeting a Resident and/or Advocate Needs to
Monitor the implementation of the care plan.
- Are the activities on the care plan done as the resident agreed?
- Is the plan meeting the resident's needs and the plan's goals?

Talk with facility staff about the implementation.
- If things are going well, let the staff know.
- If there are problems, discuss them with the staff to see what can be done.
- If adjustments aren't satisfactory to the resident or if the resident experiences some major changes, ask for another care plan meeting.

What If There are Problems?

If there are problems with the care plan or with its implementation, residents and family members can take action. In chapter 7, "Problem Solving: Being Your Own Advocate," you will learn more about how to get problems resolved. Because the care plan is recorded with measurable points, it lends itself to review and revision if implementation falls short of the plan's promise.

When problems arise, you and your loved one should:

Talk with staff about the problems and ask how they can be resolved. It's a good idea to keep notes about what you see, request, and do. Write down names, dates, and times. (See "Who's Who on the Staff" on page 4.)

Ask for another care plan meeting so everyone involved with care delivery can sit together and jointly discuss possible solutions.

Let the staff know what you want to discuss. Ask for specific staff to be present if their knowledge or agreement is important to the issue you want to discuss. Remember that nurse assistants may be helpful.

Keep the discussion focused on solving the problem, not on placing blame.

Know what you want the outcome to be before going into the meeting.

Ask for a reassessment and another care planning meeting if the resident's condition has changed in a permanent way, more than a short-term illness, for example.

Ask a long-term care ombudsman to assist you in getting your relative's needs met.

File a formal complaint with the state nursing home regulatory agency **if necessary.** (A state-by-state list appears in Appendix 7.)

Playing a Part in the Process

Resident assessment and care planning present a path for nursing home residents (and/or their advocates/family members) to be directly involved in making decisions about their care and daily life in the facility. Assessment and care planning guide facility staff in providing care that meets the individual resident's unique needs. Because these procedures are basic to everything that happens in the nursing home, they are discussed or referred to throughout this book.

For these procedures to work well, you must lend your assistance. It is often only with your motivation and support that residents are willing to actively participate in planning their care. Your voice may be needed for the resident's perspective to be included.

Immediately following this chapter, you'll find a case example that illustrates the process in detail.

If you're wondering how you can know what questions to ask about medical care, read the next chapter, "The Seven Most Common Problems in Care." It tells you how to identify good care and what to do if there are problems in a number of areas. The tips in chapter 4 will help you know what to consider when discussing your relative's care plan.

— All laws are subject to change. Regardless of any changes in the federal law discussed in this chapter, these standards are supported in some state laws as well as professional codes of conduct. They are good practice! They represent good care! As a family member you have every right to ask for and expect these practices for your relative. —

The Resident Assessment Process and Care Planning: An Example

An Overview

As you know, the key to achieving quality care for residents is the resident assessment and care planning process. Through an assessment, staff gather information about a resident's life, functioning and needs. This information is used to develop a plan of care focusing on the resident's needs. The resident and family help staff develop this plan. With a proper assessment and care plan that is carried out, the resident receives needed restorative and maintenance services. The result can be a dramatic improvement in a resident's condition.

Still Learning

All facilities are required, by the Nursing Home Reform Law, to provide care to attain or maintain the highest well-being of each resident through use of the assessment and care planning process. Assessment and care planning are an accepted standard of practice. Some facilities are still learning how to conduct assessments and prepare individualized care plans. They're also still figuring out how to help residents and families fully participate in these. Increasingly, consumers like yourself are using assessment and care planning as a forum to ask questions, discuss problems with the care, and identify possible solutions.

The Complete Assessment Process

To help you participate, one example — "Mr. Zentoff" — is followed through the entire process: from the assessment to the care plan. You'll see how Mr. Zentoff's care changes as a result of assessment and care planning. A sample section from the standard assessment form, called the Minimum Data Set (MDS)*, appears on page 53, to show the sort of information staff will be gathering and reviewing regarding your relative.

As mentioned in chapter 3, the form (MDS) is only one part of the assessment. It leads staff to dig deeper by asking more questions to understand why certain conditions exist. This digging deeper process, or further analysis, is guided by Resident Assessment Protocols (RAPs). In this section, you'll see how the RAPs add to the information on the form (MDS) and help with care planning.

Meet Mr. Zentoff

Mr. Zentoff moves into the nursing home and staff begin to get to know him by asking him and his daughter questions and by observing his abilities. Staff also look at his medical records. This process helps staff complete an assessment form called the MDS. During this process staff learn a lot about Mr. Zentoff.

Mr. Dennis Zentoff, a widower, was admitted to Shady Hill Nursing Facility with diagnoses of diabetes, Alzheimer's disease and a history of high blood pressure. He is eighty years old. He needs assistance with eating, toileting, bathing and has poor balance. The poor balance puts him at risk of falling. He receives a laxative as needed and medicine for high blood pressure.

Mr. Zentoff was a fireman on the evening shift for thirty-two years. After his retirement he kept the same schedule as during his working life. He goes to bed at one o'clock in the morning and gets up at nine a.m. He's used to snacking all day because his meal times never coordinated with his family's when his children were growing up. He has a daughter. His son died twenty years ago. Since his wife died soon after his retirement, he kept to his work day schedule.

He learned to control his diabetes even on that schedule by balancing food, insulin and exercise. For the past eight years he has gotten up at night to go to the bathroom. Otherwise he sleeps well. He was involved in the local boy's club, helping those less fortunate children in his

---

*To obtain a copy of the MDS and a two-page guide, "Assessment and Care Planning: The Key to Good Care," contact The National Citizens' Coalition for Nursing Home Reform, 1424 16th St. N.W., Suite 202, Washington, DC 20036-2211 Phone (202) 332-2275, www.nursinghomeaction.org

neighborhood. He suffers some loss of recent memory which makes it dangerous for him to remain alone. His daughter visits him every week.

You can see how much information about all aspects of Mr. Zentoff's life is collected during an assessment! From this process, staff receive information about Mr. Zentoff's past which help them adapt the facility's routines and environment to support Mr. Zentoff's functioning. By supporting Mr. Zentoff's functioning, staff will also be supporting his quality of life, as you will read in chapter 6.

Wandering Becomes an Issue

While staff are gathering the assessment information, they see Mr. Zentoff wandering around at night. Concerned about his safety, they ask his physician for a sleeping medication. This does make him sleep but his daughter is asking why he seems anxious and lethargic for the first time in his life.

On the MDS form, staff note that Mr. Zentoff walks around the facility at night by marking the MDS under Section E, Mood and Behavior Patterns. Under E-4 Behavioral Symptoms, the staff codes his wandering with a 3 to indicate he wanders daily or more frequently. This triggers staff to look at the Behavioral Symptoms RAP.

If you were Mr. Zentoff's child, you would have questioned the sleeping medication. You'll learn from the information in chapter 5 that sleeping medications are usually restraints. To see how the assessment process guided the staff to discover why Mr. Zentoff wandered all night, read on!

Sample Section of Minimum Data Set (MDS) Form

SECTION E. MOOD AND BEHAVIOR PATTERNS

4. BEHAVIORAL SYMPTOMS	(A) *Behavioral symptom frequency in last 7 days* 0. Behavior not exhibited in last 7 days 1. Behavior of this type occurred 1 to 3 days in last 7 days 2. Behavior of this type occurred 4 to 6 days, but less than daily 3. Behavior of this type occurred daily (B) *Behavioral symptom alterability in last 7 days* 0. Behavior not present OR behavior was easily altered 1. Behavior was not easily altered		
		(A)	(B)
	a. WANDERING (moved with no rational purpose, seemingly oblivious to needs or safety	*3*	*1*
	b. VERBALLY ABUSIVE BEHAVIORAL SYMPTOMS (others were threatened, screamed at, cursed at)		
	c. PHYSICALLY ABUSIVE BEHAVIORAL SYMPTOMS (others were hit, shoved, scratched, sexually abused)		
	d. SOCIALLY INAPPROPRIATE/DISRUPTIVE BEHAVIORAL SYMPTOMS (made disruptive sounds, noisiness, screaming, self-abusive acts, sexual behavior or disrobing in public, smeared/threw food/feces, hoarding, rummaged through others' belongings)		
	e. RESISTS CARE (resisted taking medications/injections, ADL assistance, or eating		

Digging Deeper with the Resident Assessment Protocol (RAP)

Each RAP contains three sections of content. Here's how the Behavioral Symptoms RAP would help staff examine Mr. Zentoff's wandering.

I. Problem: describes key characteristics of the problem condition and how this condition affects nursing home residents.

For Mr. Zentoff, staff see that Section I of the Behavioral Symptoms RAP describes the potential dangers of "wandering behavior" and explains why it's important not to use physical and chemical restraints but to find individualized approaches to address "behaviors."

II. Triggers: alert staff to the resident's potential problems or needs. Triggers guide staff in reviewing the parts of the MDS that trigger the RAP. This section describes symptoms to help staff determine if the resident needs further assessment in this problem area. Triggers relate symptoms to possible causes!

Section II triggers the staff to look at the potential link between medications and behaviors and guides the staff to look for underlying causes and possible solutions.

III. Guidelines: facilitate an assessment of factors that may cause or contribute to the triggered condition. The Guidelines also suggest potential interventions to address the problem.

Section III asks staff to observe the behavior to determine any patterns and to review potential causes of the behavior. Staff knew that Mr. Zentoff's wandering occurred at night. A sleeping pill had been prescribed for this reason before the assessment was completed. Since this RAP asks about changes in familiar routines, staff talked with Mr. Zentoff and his daughter about specific aspects of his daily routine prior to admission. The staff also reviewed the information on the entire MDS, checking for information that might be related to Mr. Zentoff's wandering during the night. If staff can determine how to restore some of Mr. Zentoff's familiar routines, he would no longer need the medication or "behave" in ways that concern staff for his safely.

It's through the RAPs that the process of trial and error begins as the assessment team seeks to determine potential causes of conditions that were identified on the MDS. Once the causes are known, solutions can begin. *Thus, the RAPs are the primary link between the MDS and care planning.*

By the time a RAP is completed, the facility should have information and ideas for addressing the need identified on the care plan. If the review of the RAP indicates a potential for rehabilitation or that a resident is at risk for developing a problem, staff can pick up some ideas to help from the RAP.

The RAPs are also an educational resource for staff and consumers. You might use the RAPs to learn what the facility needs to consider in understanding your relative's condition. The RAPs can give you ideas for approaches to suggest in care planning. The staff, or the ombudsman, can get you the RAPs if you want to read one or more of them yourself. The MDS and RAPs are also available via the Internet on the Centers for Medicare and Medicaid Services web site, http://www.hcfa.gov. So, how does this assessment information lead to a care plan? How is this information used on Mr. Zentoff's care plan?

Developing Mr. Zentoff's Care Plan

Look at one example from Mr. Zentoff's care plan: *the need to maintain his ability to walk independently in spite of his unsteadiness on his feet.* Staff put a great deal of thought and discussion into identifying the problem and developing individualized approaches to keep Mr. Zentoff walking independently. The problem identification and the approaches are based on information obtained during the assessment process. Mr. Zentoff's *customary routine* as well as his *preferences* were used to *individualize* the care plan and to guide staff in adapting to his needs.

Mr. Zentoff was included in the care planning process. He indicated to the nurse assistant that he felt adrift in the institution and didn't know what to do with himself. The staff suggested a care planning goal of keeping him safely mobile. Mr. Zentoff agreed with this goal, saying he wanted to be as independent as possible. At the care planning meeting a number of options were discussed including gardening, exercise classes, a walking program or rounds with the security force. He chose the rounds with security; he could use his keen eye to look for fires.

An *interdisciplinary team* was used. A physical therapist was asked to assess Mr. Zentoff's mobility in order to strengthen his unsteady gait and to provide for daily exercise. The therapist decided Mr. Zentoff didn't need therapy but that he did need to be encouraged to walk daily. Thus, Mr. Zentoff went on rounds with the security guard. The latter decision was made with input from the activities director, the nurse, the social worker, physical therapist, nurse assistant on the evening shift, the security guard, and Mr. Zentoff.

Including the *nurse assistant* in the care planning discussion was a key ingredient in the team's ability to develop a successful care plan. Outside of relatives and friends, the evening nurse assistant was the person who knew Mr. Zentoff best. Usually it's the day aide, but Mr. Zentoff was a night owl, so the evening assistant was included. She was the one who knew what his job had been and realized that putting him to bed at 8:00 would be traumatic and against his lifelong habit. Nurse assistants on all shifts were consulted to identify strengths and needs occurring throughout the twenty-four hour period.

If you're wondering what a care plan looks like, see the example below. The care plan might look different in your relative's nursing home because different facilities have various kinds of forms they use for care plans. The form is not important: the information on the form is very important. The care plans in all nursing homes should contain the elements described in the next section. Look how clear Mr. Zentoff's plan for walking is.

Mr. Zentoff's Care Plan for Walking

Need: Maintain Mr. Zentoff's ability to walk

Goal	Approaches	Disciplines	Re-evaluation
Mr. Zentoff will walk the length of the building three times at least five days a week.	Walk on evening rounds with security guard on all three floors at least five times a week. Security guard and Mr. Z. will report to evening nurse assistant.	Nursing Security guards Activities Physical therapy	October 25 (2 weeks)

Elements of This Care Plan

- The care plan *need* is to maintain current functioning. It has a prevention focus.
- The *goal* is specific, measurable and written in a way that anyone can understand.
- The *approach* shows respect for the resident. It's individualized and reflects ideas from many disciplines. The actual days on which Mr. Zentoff is to walk are not specified because he should have choice and flexibility. He might want to walk more often than five times a week. It is clearly the responsibility of the evening nurse assistant to see that the walk is accomplished.
- *Disciplines* (operating departments) involved are spelled out in the plan.
- The date for *re-evaluation* is clear.

Other facilities would individualize Mr. Zentoff's care plan in the following way.*

Need	**Goal**	**Approaches**
I need to walk.	I will walk the length of the building three times at least five days a week.	I am used to working at night. The security guard will ask me to walk on rounds with him every evening. I can help him check all three floors of the building. I will be watching for fires on our rounds. We will report to the evening nurse assistant who works with me.

Individualized Care

As a result of the resident assessment process and care planning, Mr. Zentoff receives care tailored to meet his needs and compatible with his lifelong routines and preferences. His care plan guides the staff in assisting him as described below.

Nurse assistants cue him to eat, dress, bathe, and use the toilet before retiring as he has always done. He goes to bed at his customary time and gets up late, missing breakfast. He gets his protein and vegetables at meal times and fills in the rest of his food in divided amounts during the day and evening. He takes only insulin and blood pressure medicines. He doesn't require sleeping pills or laxatives. He gets up, with the assistance of a nurse assistant, to use the bathroom at night. He spends his days socializing with other residents and the staff. Mr. Zentoff goes on evening rounds with the security staff.

---

* Adapted from a model developed by Susan Misiorski and Lynn MacLean, Apple Health Care, Inc., Avon, Connecticut.

Chapter 4

The Seven Most Common Problems in Care — How Can You Help?

- **Step Up** — Be observant about your relative's condition and well-being.

  - **Speak Up** — When little things don't seem right — speak up to **prevent** poor care.

    - **Advocate for Good Care** — Be sure your relative is toileted, given fluids, assisted with eating, gets good skin care, gets moved, and receives support for remaining independent.

THIS CHAPTER WILL HELP YOU DECIDE WHETHER YOUR relative is receiving good care. In the preceding chapter on assessment and care planning you learned how staff gather information about your relative to use in planning care. You also learned about your role in giving information, asking questions, and suggesting approaches. Reading this chapter will help you know what to question and will give you some ideas for suggestions you can make about care.

Nursing home staff generally try to give good individualized care, but there can be slip ups even in the better homes. Your job is to let staff know when you think good care isn't being provided. *(Don't forget to compliment those who give good care!)* Good homes will welcome your comments and suggestions. If you sense that your relative and others in the nursing home are not getting good care, let the alarm bells ring! You're probably right. Don't let the matter drop. Trust your judgement and intervene!

It's Important to Know Good Standards of Care

Good standards of care for nursing home residents are common sense. And, these common sense standards are often found in federal or state laws or regulations.

Nursing homes must provide care and services to:

- help each resident maintain everything she is able to do at admission to the home and
- reach a better level if possible.

— Good standards of care for nursing home residents are common sense. —

This means that if Mrs. Jessup's left leg and arm can be moved by staff easily on admission day, she shouldn't lose that ability during her stay in the nursing home. There are only three reasons for a resident's ability in any area to decline after admission:

- progression of a disease,
- onset of a new disease or condition, or
- a decision to refuse treatment.

Staff usually provide preventive and restorative care and residents get better. *Usually*, but not *always*. Sometimes there are not enough staff or they are poorly supervised by nurses (RN or LPN/LVN). What if Mrs. Jessup entered a nursing home without good care? Put yourself in the role of her relative. How would you know if Mrs. Jessup's decline in movement ability was due to insufficient care or due to one of the three reasons just stated?

You notice that Mrs. Jessup's movement in her left arm and leg aren't what they were before admission. When you ask questions, staff say, "It's normal for Mrs. Jessup to lose the use of her left arm and leg. After all, she had a stroke that affected her left side."

But you know that Mrs. Jessup was in the hospital after her stroke *before* she came to the nursing home. You remember that the hospital nurses moved her left arm and leg daily. In fact, her leg and arm were improving. Now in the nursing home, her arm and leg are becoming stiff and unable to be moved at all.

Think about the three reasons for unavoidable decline.

- *progression of a disease*

Mrs. Jessup's loss of function in her arm and leg isn't occurring because of disease progression. In fact, she was getting better after her stroke.

- *onset of a new disease or condition*

It isn't a new disease or condition such as pneumonia or a broken leg that is making her lose function.

- *a decision to refuse treatment*

Mrs. Jessup is eager to get better and accepts treatment.

Her loss of function is happening because the staff are not moving her left arm and leg to keep them limber. She's getting poor care. Family must step in and help Mrs. Jessup get good care.

☞ TIP: Appendix 6B, "How Do You Know When Preventive Care Is Needed?," tells you what kind of conditions put residents at risk for decline. Use these guidelines to see if your relative is at risk and what type of care prevents bad things from happening.

How Do You Know If Care is Good or Not so Good?

- *Know the extent to which improvement or recovery is possible* for Mrs. Jessup. Even though Mrs. Jessup had a stroke resulting in an immediate loss of function, the real question is how much function can she regain? Ask her doctor.

- *What are realistic rehabilitation goals* for Mrs. Jessup? Some physicians are better at estimating recovery and planning care than others. You might want a second opinion. A physical therapist can also evaluate rehabilitation potential.

- *Know the medications she is taking and how they are affecting her rehabilitation.* For instance, Mrs. Jessup may be on a drug to lower her blood pressure. That same drug may cause her to become dizzy when she stands up. Pharmacists specialize in knowing dosages, side effects and interactions of different drugs. Ask staff for a list of the drugs she's taking, plus a list of her diagnoses. Take these to a trusted pharmacist for advice. If changes are necessary, you or the pharmacists should talk to the doctor.

- Most important, *what does the resident want?* Mrs. Jessup wants to stand up again without assistance and walk with assistance, just as she had prior to her stroke. Staff might assume that because of her age and other infirmities, she wouldn't want to try rehabilitation. You learned in chapter 3, residents, families and staff should set goals *together* during care planning meetings.

Even though you may not be a nurse, physician, or social worker, you will know when your relative's care is good and when it isn't. Let's look at a list of the most common problems.

Bad Things Happen Without Good Care

1.) *Not being taken to the bathroom according to individualized needs leads to incontinence* (wet and soiled.)

2.) *Not getting enough fluids to drink leads to dehydration* (often thirsty, and very dry skin.)

3.) *Not getting enough to eat leads to malnutrition* (weight loss and cracks in the corners of the mouth.)

4.) *Not being groomed properly leads to poor hygiene* (body odors, dirty mouth.)

5.) *Not receiving preventive skin care leads to pressure sores* (holes in the skin and sometimes the muscle underneath.)

6.) *Not being helped with range of motion exercises or physical therapy leads to contractures.* (shortened muscles.)

7.) *No encouragement to retain independence leads to loss of ability to eat, dress, walk, bathe, and get in and out of bed* (increased dependency.)

Real-Life Examples of The Seven Most Common Problems...and Tips on What To Do

(In addition to the information in this section, you can gain more tips by reading Appendix 6 — "Good Care Prevents Poor Outcomes," "How Do You Know When Preventive Care Is Needed?" and "Rehabilitative and Restorative Care to Increase Function."

1.) Not being taken to the bathroom when the resident needs to go leads to incontinence.

You find your mother wet when you visit her. While you may be angry, first stop and ask yourself a few questions. Have you ever found her wet before? If the answer is no, then simply ask the staff to help clean and dry her. But if this is a common occurrence, you must take action.

Ask yourself these questions:

- How often do you find her wet?
- Does she smell?
- Examine her buttocks or clothes; have dried urine or feces been there for awhile?
- Has she only begun wetting herself recently? Have staff checked her for infection in the bladder? Are there enough staff to toilet her?

How do you know if help is needed and whether it's available:
- Can your mother get to the toilet herself? If not, does anyone help her?
- Does she know when she needs to go to the bathroom? If not, does someone remind her?
- Are staff following her own lifelong schedule of going to the bathroom?
- When do you usually find her wet?

What should you do?
- Share your findings with staff:

  Your mother is nearly always wet when you come in. She smells. There is a ring of dried urine on her clothes. Your mother needs help to get to the toilet. At home, she went to the bathroom about every three hours. You notice staff only toilet her when she asks.
- Ask staff how they will help your mother.

  Staff should help her to the toilet according to her needs, rather than their schedule. Thus, they might check with her every three hours to see if she needs assistance in toileting.
- Watch for signs to be sure staff do what they say they will. Your mother should not smell or be wet when you visit. If she is, then call for a careplanning conference. At the meeting, request a written plan indicating how staff will help your mother regain continence. Decide when you will meet again to assess their progress.

2.) Not getting enough fluids leads to dehydration.

The facility calls you one day to say that your father is going to the hospital. He has a fever. You meet him at the emergency room. The doctor says he's dehydrated, from not getting enough to drink. The doctor warns that he'll wind up in the hospital again unless he receives more fluids each day.

Sometimes dehydration is the first clue a family member has that a resident is not receiving quality care. It is easily prevented by ensuring that residents drink about ten cups of fluid a day. As your father's advocate, you know you must take action on his behalf.

Ask yourself these questions:
During the past few weeks, were there any of the following signs of dehydration?

- Did your father's mouth look dry?
- Did his tongue stick to the inside of his mouth?
- Did his lips appear dry; maybe even peeling slightly?
- Did his skin look or feel drier than usual?
- Did his eyes look sunken?

How do you know if help is needed and whether it's available:
- Does your father remember how to drink? Is he receiving help?
- What is his favorite drink? When and where does he like to have it? Is that happening?
- Is there always something available to drink?
- Does he drink everything on his tray at mealtime?
- Does he seem to crave a drink when you visit?
- Does he take medication that might cause dehydration such as a diuretic that makes him urinate often?
- Does he act a little more confused than usual? (Dehydration is a cause of confusion in older people.)
- Does his urine smell strong?

What should you do?
- Share your findings with the staff:
  Looking back, you might find that your father's mouth, lips and skin looked dry recently. He wasn't able to drink by himself. He drank everything you offered him. He was not on any medications that made him urinate more. He did seem very confused. In fact, you had mentioned it to the staff previously.
- Ask how staff plan to help your father.
  Staff should be able to tell you they will offer your father his favorite beverage, who will be responsible for helping him to drink it, and when he will be offered it. They should ensure that your father is getting enough to drink.
- Watch for signs to be sure staff do what they say they will.
  Visit your father at different times of the day. If you suspect that he's becoming dehydrated again, ask for a care planning conference. At the meeting, work out a schedule that addresses what he will get to drink, when it will be offered to him, and who will be in charge of getting it to him. Follow up by visiting at different times and monitoring whether your father's skin, mouth and eyes look moist, as they should. Dehydration should not occur again.

3.) Not getting enough to eat leads to malnutrition.
Your daughter comes home from college for a visit and drops in on
her grandmother at the nursing home. Your daughter, who hasn't
seen her grandmother since she entered the home three months ago,
is astonished to find that her grandmother has lost so much weight.
When she mentions it, you realize something has been bothering
you about your mother, but you didn't know exactly what. You feel
terrible, but sensibly stop to ask a few important questions.

You ask yourself:
- Do your mother's clothes fit loosely?
- Are there cracks around her mouth?
- Do her lips and mouth look pale?
- Has she complained that her false teeth no longer fit?
- When do you think she began losing weight?
- Does she appear confused?
- Is her skin breaking down?

How do you know if help is needed and whether it's available:
- Can your mother feed herself? If not, does someone help her?
- What is her favorite meal of the day? Is it served when and where
  she wants it? Does she take a long time to eat? Is she rushed
  through meals? Is she assisted with eating until she's full?
- Does she seem uninterested in food? Do staff know why?
- Does she like the food ? Can she choose from a menu?
- Has staff told you she is losing weight? Have they asked for
  your help?
- Have staff routinely weighed your mother?

What should you do?
- Share what you found with staff.
  Looking back, you find that your mother's clothes do look
  baggy and she appears smaller sitting in her favorite chair she
  brought from home. She always eats well when you are there,
  but it does take an hour to help her eat. She has always
  enjoyed mealtime, and loves the foods you bring from home.
  You notice she turns her head to the side when she swallows.
  Her lips and mouth are pale.
- Ask for a care planning conference immediately.
  You should have been told about your mother's weight loss.
  Find out what staff know about your mother's weight loss.
  Have they assessed her for depression and for swallowing

problems – common causes of not eating? Work with the staff and your mother to develop a care plan. Your mother might need food more frequently and in smaller amounts. The plan should include your mother's meal plan, how it will be served, and who will assist her at each meal. (Lack of staff is a major cause of malnutrition in nursing homes.) You may want to help by continuing to bring her favorite foods to the nursing home. Loss of appetite and weight loss can indicate depression. Staff should assess your mother for depression which is treatable with good results.

- Monitor your mother to see that she gets the care she needs. You should see a weight gain and the signs of malnutrition should disappear. Be sure to attend the next care planning conference so that you, your mother, and the staff can evaluate her progress together.

4.) Not being groomed properly leads to poor hygiene. Your mother was discharged from the hospital very quickly after a hip replacement. She was admitted to a nursing home recommended by the hospital social worker. After the first week, you become very worried because your mother appears disheveled. Her mouth smells and looks dirty. There is a heavy, stale odor coming from her body. You angrily wonder why the social worker suggested this nursing home to you. You know you must do something.

Ask yourself these questions:

- Is your mother the only one in the nursing home you see in this condition?
- How many others appear the way she does?
- Are other family members worried? Has the family council (see chapter 7) worked on this issue?
- Do the staff seem harried, unable to complete their work?
- Do staff sit at the nurses' desk unoccupied, or watch television?
- Does your mother have a clean washcloth and towel?
- Is her toothbrush wet in the mornings and evenings indicating use?
- What can your mother tell you about the situation?
- What care does she receive on evenings and weekends?

After talking with other families, you learn the hospital social worker recommends this nursing home, not knowing what the care is like. It is the community's only nursing home. Other residents and family members share your dissatisfaction. The administrator and director of nursing say Medicaid doesn't reimburse the home enough to give better care. Staff are distressed. They confide they would like something done.

What should you do?

- Contact the ombudsman and licensing and certification agency. Contact a citizen advocacy group if there is one. Information about these is in chapter 7, "Problem Solving: Being Your Own Advocate." Lists telling you how to contact them are in Appendix 7 and on the Internet site, www.nursinghomeaction.org.

  If possible, ask other families to join you.

- You may find that neither the ombudsman nor licensing and certification officials are successful in getting the nursing home to change.

  In this case, you must request federal investigators to intervene and conduct a survey. (Contact information is listed at the end of Appendix 7.) You might also contact the home's owners or corporate headquarters or your legislators or congressional representatives.

- Legal counsel and other recourses may be in order. A citizen advocacy group or the National Citizens' Coalition for Nursing Home Reform may be able to help you. You may need to find a lawyer to represent you.

A call to the local press is another option to consider. Sometimes concerned editors and reporters take an interest in alerting the community to a story of poor care in a neighborhood nursing home.

5.) No preventive skin care leads to pressure sores

Your father always loves to have his back rubbed. One day you notice a little break in his skin right at the end of his backbone. You report it to the nurse. A week later when you give him a back rub, you discover a bandage on the skin break. Your father appeared to wince when you rubbed near it. You ask the nurse about it. She says they're treating it. You're concerned, but try to collect yourself and assess the situation before taking further action.

What you need to know about pressure sores:
- Pressure sores usually are preventable.
- Poor nutrition, insufficient fluids, unclean skin, and the inability to move without help increase the chance that a pressure sore will develop.

Ask yourself these questions:
- Is your father left sitting in his own urine or feces?
- Is he getting enough to drink?
- Is he eating properly?
- Is he unable to move and reposition himself without help?

How do you know if help is needed and if it is available?
- You have already learned what to ask about incontinence, dehydration, and malnutrition which could explain the first three observations in the preceding list.

If your father is unable to move himself, ask:
- Do staff get him out of bed, into a chair every day? Is his chair comfortable?
- Do they turn or reposition him often enough to prevent sores?

What should you do?
- Share with staff what you know.

  Your father isn't able to move by himself very well anymore. He sits in a chair for long periods during the day. He rarely changes positions when he's in bed. He drinks and eats well. Every now and then he soils himself. He says sometimes the night staff are so busy they don't answer his bell when he needs to go to the bathroom.
- Ask staff how they will cure the sore at the end of his backbone and prevent future pressure sores.

  The sores are forming because your father is remaining in one place for long periods of time. Thus, staff should come up with a schedule for moving or repositioning your father at least every two hours. He should not lie on his back at all while the sore heals. You should be told approximately when your father will be repositioned and by whom.
- Monitor your father's care.

  Visit at various times, even late at night, to see that your father is being turned as promised. The sore on his backbone should heal within a reasonable period of time, and no new sores should develop.

6.) No range of motion exercises leads to contractures
Your Great Aunt Maude, who has Alzheimer's disease, entered a nursing home six months ago when her family could no longer take care of her. This is your first visit. You are shocked to find her in bed, curled up like a baby. She recognizes you, but is unable to move and is being fed by a tube in her nose. You learn that the nurses have told her family that many older people get this way, and that it can't be helped. You are determined to do something.

Ask yourself these questions:
- Do staff get Aunt Maude up every day?
- When did she stop walking?
- Why is she being fed through a feeding tube?
- Has her family met with the staff and doctor?
- What does Maude say about her care?
  The staff tell you that Aunt Maude came to the nursing home after she could no longer walk. She got up every day and enjoyed her meals. Aunt Maude has never complained in the nursing home.
  You know Aunt Maude and her family are trusting people. They accept what the staff have told them that it was better that Aunt Maude stay in bed. Her family didn't realize she couldn't move her legs and arms. They thought she curled up because she was most comfortable that way. The staff told the family there wasn't a reason to call Aunt Maude's physician because there hasn't been any change in her condition.

How do you know if help is needed and whether she is getting the help?
- Do staff help her move all her joints in every direction every day?
- Do they use pillows and cushions to help her sit comfortably?
- Do they do use pillows so that she lies straight in the bed?

What should you do?
- Your aunt has suffered permanent damage.
  You and her family must immediately report this incident of gross neglect to the local Long Term Care Ombudsman and to the licensing and certification agency. If those agencies are unable to help, contact a citizen advocacy group if there is one. Contact information for these agencies and groups is in Appendix 7 and on the Internet at www.nursinghomeaction.org.

Aunt Maude has received extremely poor care. Contractures are almost always preventable with daily range-of-motion exercises. These exercises are usually done with the help of a nurse aide. Each joint is carefully moved in every range of motion possible, starting with the neck and moving down the body to the toes.

This movement keeps joints mobile and muscles stretched. Muscles that are not stretched become contracted. Aunt Maude's condition graphically illustrates the truism, "If you don't use it, you'll lose it." Although intensive physical therapy may help, irreversible harm has occurred. The contractures will cause Aunt Maude discomfort the rest of her life. Her arms are tight to her body; her heels touch her buttocks. These are the consequences of serious and unacceptable neglect.

• Consider taking Aunt Maude to another facility.
If that isn't possible, you must try to get the home she's in to start giving the best care possible!

• Request to speak with the physician.
Find out why no one ordered therapy. If the physician appears negligent, contact the physicians' licensing board in your state.

• Ask Aunt Maude if she would agree to have another physician see her.
If she agrees, you should be there when the new doctor visits. Ask the new physician how the staff should care for the contractures.

• Call for a care planning conference.
Try to arrange to have an ombudsman or other advocate accompany you. Nursing home staff may be defensive under the circumstances.

During the meeting, carefully ask questions about the need for a feeding tube. In facilities that give poor care, a feeding tube may be used simply for staff's convenience. If the tube can be removed, Aunt Maude may derive some enjoyment from eating regular food once again. Also find out how staff will prevent pressure sores since Aunt Maude can no longer move herself. What exactly will they do? Who will do it? When will it be done?

- Arrange a schedule with Aunt Maude's relatives to visit her often and at various times.
  Visitors should monitor every aspect of Aunt Maude's care, from who's seeing that her skin is being cared for properly, what and how she's eating and drinking, to when she's being repositioned.
- Using the family council, alert other families about the poor care Aunt Maude received.
  Remind them to ensure that whatever joints a resident is able to move should remain flexible. Advise them to urge staff to provide range-of-motion exercises and other preventive and rehabilitative measures to prevent stiff joints from developing into contractures.

7.) No encouragement to retain independence leads to loss of ability to eat, dress, walk, bathe, and get in and out of bed.
Your father worked hard to learn to dress himself again after his stroke. He still needed help getting his clothes out of the closet. And, once the clothes were out of the closet, he approached them at his own, slow pace. Those stumbling blocks, however, were largely eclipsed by the immense satisfaction he derived from remastering these basic steps to independence.

He still can't talk very well and has a hard time getting his words out. So it's not surprising that he hasn't told you that a new nurse wouldn't let him dress and groom himself because, she said, it took him too long. He couldn't make himself understood and finally gave up trying to explain that he preferred to handle the task himself. Meanwhile, you find it puzzling that he let his beard grow. You suspect something is going on.

Ask yourself these questions
- Is it your father's choice to let his beard grow?
- Is he wearing his clothes the way he would prefer?
- Does he wear his favorite clothes?

How do you know if help is needed and whether it's available?
- Is staff helping your father be independent, or taking a short cut and doing things for him?
- Does he get dressed when he has the most energy?
- Are staff trying to understand him?
  A person who has regained the ability to dress and groom himself should continue to be able to do it. Your father could

understand but couldn't make himself understood. Staff were neither taking the time to communicate with him nor helping his family communicate with him.

What should you do?

- If your father can see and read, try communicating with him through writing.

  Ask him if he wants the beard. If he does not, tell the staff.

- Ask whether a speech therapist has been consulted.

  If there has been a consultation, find out what the therapist planned for care. If there has been no consultation, request one.

- Find out when the next care planning conference is scheduled, and say you want to attend.

  If no conference has been planned, ask that one be arranged. Attend, with your father, prepared to ask questions about his speech and how you can work together to help staff understand him better. Develop a plan with your father and staff that encourages him to dress and shave at his own speed.

- Monitor the situation to see that staff carry out the plan.

From Good to Bad to Worse — Now What?

Certain problems will prove easier to correct than others. As you noticed, each of these examples of common problems was more complicated than the previous one. That doesn't mean loss of independence is more or less difficult to solve than dehydration. The range of situations shows you that usually it's easy to work with staff to solve a problem. But, sometimes it isn't. Think about solving problems as a step-by-step process.

Work with the nursing home staff, especially through the care planning process (chapter 3), to promote needed rehabilitation programs and restorative services. See Appendix 6C.

- Look for evidence that staff are carrying out both preventive and restorative programs.
- Ask questions if you discover preventive or rehabilitative programs are not occurring as promised.
- Check with other residents and families in the nursing home to see whether they are receiving these programs and services.
- Use the family council as a resource if other residents have the same problems.

- Use outside sources if necessary including ombudsman program, regulatory systems, state licensing and certification agencies, and federal government agencies (chapter 7).
- Use citizen advocacy groups, the press, and as a last resort, legal action. Legal action is costly and slow.

Step Up, Speak Out, and Advocate for Good Care

Staff try to give good care, but sometimes, for a variety of reasons they don't. Then, you have to act.

Ask yourself these questions about your relative's care and write down the answers.

- What signs and symptoms do you see?
- What kind of help does he need?
- Is he getting the assistance he needs? Are there enough staff?

After collecting the information in writing, then:

- share your findings with the staff
- ask how, and in what time frame, they plan to respond to your information
- if they do not give you their plan in writing, write it down yourself
- be sure the plan is carried out as specified
- ask for a care planning conference when needed

  Follow-up to see that the care plan is carried out. Take additional steps to get good care if the care plan is not followed. See chapter 7 for tips on solving problems.

— All laws are subject to change. Regardless of any changes in the federal law discussed in this chapter, these standards are supported in some state laws as well as professional codes of conduct. They are good practice! They represent good care! As a family member you have every right to ask for and expect these practices for your relative. —

Chapter 5

Good Care Is Restraint-Free

- **Step Up** — Observe if people are tied up or if they seemed drugged in your nursing home.

  - **Speak Out** — if physical or chemical restraints are suggested for your relative.

    - **Advocate for Good Care** — instead of restraint use.

IN CHAPTER 4, YOU LEARNED ABOUT THE SEVEN MOST common problems in poor care. This chapter focuses on number eight. An entire chapter is devoted to the use of restraints because use is common and people have misconceptions about this practice. The real inside story on restraints may surprise you as you read the following pages! Federal law, some state laws, and standards of practice, now require that residents are to be virtually free of restraints!

If you know the issues, you can help staff understand how to provide care without using restraints. Research has shown that *restraints are dangerous and destructive.* Professional caregivers have learned how to eliminate restraints by studying the care of nursing home residents in other countries.

Unfortunately, some nursing homes have not adopted these new ways. That's why you may see residents tied to their chairs and beds (physically restrained), or looking listless and sleepy from mind-altering drugs (chemically restrained). This chapter provides the information you'll need to prevent your family member from being restrained.

This chapter uses the term, "behavioral symptoms." People who are unable to express feelings of pleasure or distress through words

— perhaps due to medical conditions such as dementia or stroke — express themselves through actions (ex. pacing, yelling). Behavioral symptoms, as we've used the term, are actions expressing distress that indicate an *unmet need*. As a family member of a resident, you play an essential role in helping staff understand the meaning of a behavioral symptom.

What are Restraints?

There are two kinds of restraints: *physical restraints* and *chemical restraints*.

Physical restraints prevent a person from moving freely. A physical restraint restricts one's ability to move or reach a part of the body. The most common forms of physical restraints are:

- Vest restraints used to tie a person to a bed or chair to prevent getting up
- Waist restraints also used to tie someone to a bed or chair
- Crotch restraints used to prevent someone from slipping out of a chair
- Wrist restraints to prevent a person from moving his arm
- Mitts, which look like boxing gloves, to prevent grasping anything or scratching
- Chairs with tray tables, roll bars, or lap cushions to prevent rising
- Sheets or other devices are if used to tie people into a bed or chair
- Bed side rails to keep a person from getting out of bed.

Bed rails are restraints when they keep someone from getting out of bed against her will. There are good uses for side rails: transporting residents in bed safely, supporting independence in turning in bed for a partially paralyzed individual, and supporting someone as she gets out of bed. Yet bed rails can cause harm and even death. Demented, frail, very old women are the most likely to be harmed. Meeting a new standard of care is difficult because the public and all health care workers have been taught that bed rails mean safety. Frail elders fall a greater distance with the bed rail up. Furthermore, deaths occur when weakened residents fall between the mattress and the bed rail and suffocate. The same approach is used to decrease bed rail use as for other restraint reduction.

Chemical restraints are psychoactive or mind-altering drugs used to control a person's behavioral symptoms (when other forms of care would be more appropriate). Psychoactive drugs act on the chemicals of the brain that affect thinking, feeling, reacting and paying attention.

Psychoactive drugs are not chemical restraints when they are used to treat severe mental illness, such as schizophrenia or a depression that does not respond to other therapies. Proper use can improve a patient's quality of life.

Psychoactive drugs include:

- Antipsychotics or major tranquilizers (to treat serious mental illness or distress)
- Sedatives/hypnotics (to treat insomnia/sleeplessness)
- Antidepressants (to treat depression)
- Anxiolytics or minor tranquilizers (to treat anxiety)
- Other drugs with psychoactive effects such as antihistamines.

Who is Most Likely to Be Restrained?

Nursing home residents most likely to be restrained are those who are older, physically frail, and likely to fall or are confused.* In nursing homes staff are really working to eliminate restraints. The number of individuals who are most likely to be restrained keeps getting smaller, because staff are learning better ways to provide care!

What are the Possible Bad Effects of Physical Restraints?

Physical restraints can cause all the physical effects of immobility, including:

- Incontinence because a restrained person cannot get to the bathroom
- Dehydration because a restrained person can't get anything to drink
- Urinary tract infections from incontinence, lack of fluids, and not moving
- Contractures because muscles and joints can't move
- Pressure sores from sitting too long
- Swollen feet and ankles from remaining in one position

---

*Evan, Lois K. & Strumpf, Neville E. (1989). "Trying Down the Elderly: A Review of the Literature on Physical Restraint," *Journal of the American Geriatrics Society.* 37: 65-74.

- Pneumonia from not moving, especially when a vest restraint is used
- Brittle bones leading to fractures from lack of use
- Malnutrition, because not moving decreases the appetite. Restrained people are sometimes too depressed to eat.
- Physical restraint use increases chemical restraint use.

Physical restraints make a person completely *dependent on others* for food, drink, toileting, and moving. Most nursing homes don't have enough staff to care for that many dependent people.

Physical restraints also pose the *risk of death* due to compression of the chest or strangulation, being caught in bed rails, or between the mattress and the side rail.

Further, physical restraint use causes many *psychological effects*, including:

- Agitation
- Screaming and yelling
- Depression
- Loneliness (staff and family spend less time with restrained residents)
- Withdrawal from other people.

Restrained residents say, "I feel like a prisoner" or "I've never been so humiliated." Other residents have asked, "Why are they punishing me?" or worry how they would escape the nursing home in the event of a fire. Still more say they feel as if their chest is being crushed, or voice frustration over not being able to use their hands or to go to the toilet at night, forcing them to wet their bed. Others simply resign themselves, saying, "It must be for my own good; maybe I would fall without it."*

Residents who are unable to speak show their distress by continually pulling at their clothes and the restraint, trying to remove it. Or, they become frantic, revealing anxious faces, moving constantly or yelling out. Sometimes, families think physical and chemical restraints will protect the resident. Actually they do just the opposite.

---

*Strumpf, Neville E. & Evans, Lois K. (1988). "Physical Restraint of the Hospitalized Elderly: Perceptions of Patients and Nurses," *Nursing Research*, Vol. 37, pp. 132-137.

What are the Possible Bad Effects of Chemical Restraints?

Immobility. The same physical effects of immobility caused by physical restraints can occur when chemical restraints are used. This is because chemically restrained people may be sleepy and unresponsive, sitting in one position for long periods of time.

Repetitive movements. Some chemical restraints can also cause a resident to have repetitive movements of the head and tongue, which is known as tardive dyskinesia. These movements may not go away even when the drug is stopped.

Agitation. Sometimes, a drug intended to calm a resident has the reverse effect. The resident becomes even more agitated. Unknowing staff may then ask the physician for a larger dose, which only increases the agitation or causes death.

Too many drugs. The effects of taking many kinds of drugs, called polypharmacy, is especially dangerous for older people. For example, many drugs, including some psychoactive drugs, cause blood pressure to drop, leading to falls that may result in hip fracture. A chemical restraint increases the danger of this occurring.

After reading about the bad effects of restraints, you're probably wondering if there are any rules nursing facilities and physicians have to follow about restraints. There's good news, the answer is Yes! The restrictions on using restraints have been included in federal law and in some state laws. These laws changed the standard of practice to individualized care in place of restraints.

How Do You Know Whether Restraint Use is Right or Wrong?

Here are three rules to help you decide about the use of restraints:

- *The restraint must do more good than harm* — remember, you already know restraints cause harm.
- *If your relative is unable to consent to a restraint, then it's your decision whether to consent to the treatment.* First, you must be informed of all the potential hazards and other ways care needs can be met.
- *If a restraint is necessary, the least restrictive restraint must be used* for the shortest amount of time possible.
  Even if a physician orders a physical or chemical restraint, residents and families should always question the order especially if these three rules did not guide the decision.

Physical Restraints

Many nursing homes have eliminated all physical restraints!
Facilities are doing this because of the extensive research showing
that with restraints, the risk of
injury or death is greater than
the risk of falling and injuring
oneself without them. Always question restraint use carefully. The
only exception might be in the event of an emergency. If you're
wondering what an emergency is, read on!

— Many nursing homes have eliminated all physical restraints! —

Delirium. Sometimes older people become severely agitated or
upset and may even slip in and out of consciousness. This
condition is called *delirium.* The cause usually is an infection or a
bad reaction to a drug. This is considered an emergency. Sometimes
a physical restraint is used so that the cause of the delirium can be
found and treated. If the cause isn't found and treated, death may
result. Thus the risk of using a restraint for a short time clearly
outweighs the risk of death from untreated delirium.

Life-Sustaining Treatment. Sometimes intravenous (IV) fluids or
medications are required to treat a medical condition. A resident
might try to pull out the IV tube. It's best if a family member stays
during treatment to prevent the tube from being pulled out. If no
one is available, a mitt like a boxing glove is used to prevent a
resident from grasping the tube with the thumb and forefinger. A
mitt is the least restrictive restraint to use in this situation because
it only immobilizes the fingers, whereas a wrist restraint
immobilizes the whole arm.

Restraints are sometimes used to prevent a resident from pulling
out a naso-gastric tube. This tube, known as an NG tube, is used
for feeding. The decision to use an NG tube (or a surgically placed
peg tube that goes directly to the stomach) must be weighed
carefully. Even in this situation, diverting strategies, such as a soft
ball to squeeze in each hand may make a restraint unnecessary.
The resident's wishes, the effect on quality of life, and the short- or
long-term nature of the treatment, must be considered. It's hard to
justify an NG tube for long periods of time.

These decisions should involve the whole care team, including
the resident and her family. (Refer to chapter 3 on assessment and
care planning to see how care planning is an opportunity to
discuss treatment decisions.)

So how do you decide if physical restraint use is right or wrong? Some common situations follow. Each of these describes a situation where physical restraints were improperly used and then explains what staff would do instead, to give good care.

• **Residents with unsafe mobility/postural instability**

Poor Care, Improper Restraint Use. Mrs. Saphire, a tiny woman, is very old and frail. Her bones are brittle and she falls easily. She fidgets in the big geri-chair that has a tray table to keep her from getting up and hurting herself. The chair restrains her.

Good Care, Restraint-Free. Staff thoroughly assess Mrs. Saphire to find out why she falls. Following that, staff develop an individualized care plan that includes therapy to strengthen her muscles and bones. Mrs. Saphire gets a chair fitted to her for both comfort and safety. Staff help her move often to prevent her sitting past the point of discomfort. Staff know that many older people need to change their position very frequently.

• **Residents who wander, intrude on other residents, or try to leave the nursing home**

Poor Care, Improper Restraint Use. Every morning, Mr. Delgado tries to leave the nursing home. He's a large man with Alzheimer's disease who had been a vegetable farmer all his life. Even though he could walk when he came into the facility, staff tie him in a wheelchair with a vest restraint each day to keep him from wandering away. Staff fear that Mr. Delgado would be struck by a car in the street.

Good Care, Restraint-Free. Staff assess Mr. Delgado to learn why he tries to leave the facility every morning. They discover that he's following the rhythm of his life: leaving his house to work in the fields. The nursing home has a safe outdoor space where Mr. Delgado can continue to garden and exercise. This activity makes him feel useful, keeps him safe, and maintains his muscle strength. In addition to all of these benefits, this activity sustains Mr. Delgado's quality of life!

• **Residents who are confused and/or agitated**

Poor Care, Improper Restraint Use. Mary Lou Lisner had many little strokes that affected her brain but not her physical abilities. She is quite agitated much of the time and her judgment is poor. Sometimes she becomes so agitated that she strikes staff or other residents. She is restrained in her chair with a waist restraint. Staff say the restraint is to protect others.

Good Care, Restraint-Free. Staff assess Ms. Lisner to find out what situations cause her to become agitated. By making careful observations over a few days, they find that Ms. Lisner only becomes agitated around loud noise and activity. By turning off her television, using pagers instead of loudspeakers for staff, and keeping Ms. Lisner away from busy areas, she is no longer agitated. There is no danger to others.

- **Residents who get up at night**

Poor Care, Improper Restraint Use. Jesse Feldman gets up every night as do most older people. Staff are afraid he will injure himself, so they raise his bed rail. They don't realize that the bed rail *increases* his chance of falling as he tries to climb over it to get up.

Good Care, Restraint-Free. Staff assess Mr. Feldman to find out why he gets up at night. They learn that he's used to going to the bathroom around 2 a.m. Staff help him to the bathroom every night just before 2, thus eliminating the need for the bed-rail restraint.

Chemical Restraints

The use of psychoactive drugs is more complicated than physical restraints. Unlike a physical restraint, you cannot see a chemical restraint. In addition, psychoactive drugs that are harmful when used as restraints can be beneficial when used to treat certain kinds of mental illnesses.

Beneficial Uses. As you read in the beginning of this chapter, psychoactive drugs, under certain circumstances, can significantly improve quality of life for residents. What kind of conditions can be improved by psychoactive drugs?

- **Residents with long-term mental illness, such as schizophrenia or depression**

Mrs. Johnson saw the army coming over the hill to kill her. Although she was safe and there was no army approaching her nursing home, this thought seemed very real to her. It had plagued her for years. The right psychoactive drug removed this terrifying thought and improved her quality of life.

- **Residents with dementia, who sometimes have frightening feelings and ideas that cause them to injure themselves or other people**

Mrs. Tabor continually hit those around her. She said her father, who died years ago, told her to do it. This fearful thought was successfully treated with a psychoactive drug.

• **Residents with depression so severe that simple caring measures do not help**

Mrs. Beinstock tried to commit suicide by not eating and saving all her medications to take at one time. A psychoactive drug helped her to feel well enough to benefit from therapy and activities.

Used effectively, as described in the above situations, psychoactive drugs are not considered restraints. The benefits to the resident clearly outweigh the risk of side effects and bad outcomes from the drug. In these cases, the distressing symptoms of the disease could not be controlled without drugs. The drug *enables* the resident to function a higher level without distress.

Improper Uses. However, there are many situations in which psychoactive drugs are used improperly as chemical restraints instead of giving good care. Here are some examples:

• **Residents who resist care because they don't understand what is happening to them**

Poor Care, Improper Restraint Use. Mr. Francesco hits Jenny West, his nurse aide, when she takes him to the shower on Tuesdays and Fridays. Staff gave him a chemical restraint the doctor had ordered on bath days.

Good Care, Restraint-Free. Ms. West, the nurse aide, finds another way to make Mr. Francesco comfortable during bathing. She makes the bath routine similar to what it was at home – a sponge bath at the sink. Mr. Francesco feels secure. Thus his need to resist care is eliminated and his quality of life is maintained.

• **Residents who go into other residents' rooms or try to leave the facility because they feel as if they have something important to do**

Poor Care, Improper Restraint Use. Mrs. Jaffrey, who has Alzheimer's disease, rummages through resident and staff papers whenever she can. She had been a secretary all her life. The sight of papers makes her think she has work to do. To protect other residents and staff, a chemical restraint is ordered by her doctor.

Good Care, Restraint-Free. Staff make some papers easily accessible to her for her to organize instead of using a chemical restraint. Mrs. Jaffrey stays busily occupied. She's content and feels useful.

- **Residents who curse and hit when they become frightened**

Poor Care, Improper Restraint Use. Mrs. Fromm has recent memory loss. She also has poor hearing and eyesight. She swears and hits out at staff when they approach her from behind or from the side. Mrs. Fromm feels threatened and instinctively defends herself. A physician ordered a chemical restraint for staff safety.

Good Care, Restraint Free. Staff carefully observe Mrs. Fromm. They realize Mrs. Fromm needs to be approached slowly from the front. They know to address her in a clear, reassuring voice. Using these simple techniques works! Mrs. Fromm no longer swears and hits staff.

- **Residents who cry out or act out continually because they can't tell staff they have an unmet need**

Poor Care, Improper Restraint Use. Trevor Jackson can no longer talk. His continual moaning is very upsetting to residents and staff around him. A chemical restraint is used to keep him quiet.

Good Care, Restraint-Free. Staff try to find out what is bothering him. They assume that he's moaning for a reason. Is he suffering from pain, thirst, hunger, or fatigue? Does he need to go to the toilet? They learn that his moaning is a signal to take him to the bathroom. When they respond, Mr. Jackson stops moaning. This important piece of information is written on his care plan.

- **Residents who become upset because the environment is not supportive**

Poor Care, Improper Restraint Use. Celeste Pringle lashes out at staff when they don't let her go to bed late and get up late in the morning as she had always done at home. Staff got a doctor's order for a chemical restraint so she wouldn't hurt them.

Good Care, Restraint-Free. Staff review Ms. Pringle's "Customary Routines" on her assessment form for clues to explain her lashing out. They adjust their routines so she goes to bed and gets up according to her lifelong pattern. A drug isn't needed! Ms. Pringle's quality of life is supported.

- **Residents who become upset because they are physically restrained**

Poor Care, Improper Restraint Use. James Fountain tries to leave the facility every evening. To protect him, they asked his physician for a physical restraint order. Whenever he's restrained with a vest, Mr. Fountain becomes very upset. The physician ordered a chemical restraint to calm Mr. Fountain when he's restrained physically.

Good Care, Restraint-Free. Staff wonder why Mr. Fountain wants to leave every evening. Unable to find an immediate explanation, they decide to accompany him or engage him in some other way during that time of the evening. This approach is recorded on his care plan. Neither a physical nor a chemical restraint is needed. Mr. Fountain remains active and calm.

Why are Restraints Used?

Staff sometimes use restraints because they don't have the knowledge to assess each resident and her environment. Not knowing how to assess behavioral symptoms, staff call the physician for a restraint order.

Some physicians assume that staff have done a good assessment to find the cause of a behavioral symptom. The physician's expectation is that individualized care has been tried. Therefore, a restraint is the only option remaining.

Other physicians may not know how to care for people with behavioral symptoms without using restraints. Residents and their families must always question a chemical or physical restraint order!

What Do I Ask if Chemical or Physical Restraints are Suggested or Used?

If nursing home staff suggest or use chemical or physical restraints for your relative, it's important to ask several questions.

- *What symptom prompted use of a restraint?*
- *What is causing the symptom?*
- *What efforts been made to treat or eliminate the cause?*
- *If the cause of the symptom can't be found and eliminated, are staff using individualized care practices?*

- *What is the plan for gradually discontinuing the use of physical and/or chemical restraints?*

Let's examine each of these questions in turn, and consider how you can use them.

What symptom prompted use of a restraint? Physical restraints are used most often to prevent or control falling, wandering or agitation. Since there are other ways of providing care for these conditions, a physical restraint should not be used. Good assessment and rehabilitation are more appropriate. More information about such care practices is in the section, "Individualized Care for Common Challenges Residents Face" following this chapter.

Chemical restraints are used to treat behavioral symptoms, such as wandering, agitation, objecting to care or continuous crying out. You know from the introduction to this chapter that behavioral symptoms indicate that a person has an unmet need and is feeling distressed. Therefore, the appropriate response to identifying the unmet need is a good assessment. You might recall from chapter 3, "Assessment and Care Planning," that an assessment looks at facts and asks *Why* certain problems exist.

Behavioral Symptoms and Dementing Illnesses. Residents with dementing illnesses, such as Alzheimer's disease, often have behavioral symptoms. If you understand what it's like to have a dementing illness, you'll be able to ask better questions. You'll also be better able to make helpful suggestions about what to try.

People have described dementia as being in a foreign country, where everyone but you speaks a different language. There is no way to communicate! You begin to misunderstand what is going on around you. As a result, your behavior changes. You may lose your temper rather quickly because you feel threatened. That doesn't mean you are misbehaving; rather, it means that you are expressing your distress.

Staff Response. Staff who may not understand the nature of a dementing illness sometimes label the resident as a "behavior problem." To the contrary, these behavioral symptoms tell us what the person with dementia cannot express — that there is an undiagnosed condition or unmet need. *Here is where you can really help.* Staff and family together must find out what the need is and meet it!

Has the cause of the symptom been assessed? Individual assessment is the key to preventing the use of chemical and physical restraints. Chapter 3 discusses the importance of assessing each resident and how assessment is done. You shouldn't always assume an appropriate assessment has been carried out. You should ask the staff what they have done to assess the following:

• *Is the resident receiving a high dosage of a particular drug or too many drugs?* Older people with dementia are very sensitive to all kinds of drugs that may cause a new behavioral symptom. (Isn't this true of all older people?)

• *Is there an undiagnosed condition, such as a urinary tract infection or stroke?* Most adults know they are physically ill because they feel an ache or pain. Older people may show the same illness by a change in behavior.

• *Is poor hearing or sight causing the resident to misinterpret what goes on around him?* Older people with poor hearing and vision often withdraw or become suspicious of others.

• *Is a dementing illness causing a resident to misinterpret what people say or do or to misinterpret what is going on around her?*

• *Is the resident unable to express unmet needs, such as hunger, thirst, fatigue, mobility, getting to the bathroom, and pain?* For instance, a hungry individual may try to take food from others. Knowing that hunger is the problem and meeting this need is the solution.

• *Is there a long-standing mental illness other than dementia that needs appropriate treatment?*

Environmental assessments also are important in preventing restraint use. The social climate of the home — the way staff, residents, and families are treated — and the physical environment together must support residents' safety and independence. Staff who don't rely on restraints have

> — *The environment causes 75 percent to 90 percent of the behavioral symptoms for which restraints are ordered.* —

learned that the *environment causes 75 percent to 90 percent of the behavioral symptoms* for which restraints are ordered.

You should ask the staff what they've done to assess the way the total environment affects the resident.

• *Is each resident's care based on his lifelong habits and routines, like getting up and going to bed, getting to the toilet, snacking, eating and drinking?*

- *Do staff understand that a resident with a dementing illness has extreme difficulty adjusting to new routines and often misinterprets what goes on around him?*
- *Do staff approach residents carefully? Do staff really listen to what residents say, observe what they do, and try to understand the feelings behind a resident's words and actions?*
- *Does care take into account a resident's cultural, religious and work history?*
- *Does the facility assign staff permanently to residents to provide continuity in care on all three shifts?*
- *Do staff approach residents carefully, calmly and give care in respectful ways?*

In assessing a home's physical environment, you should ask:

- *Does the home have restorative programs that promote independent and safe walking, eating, getting to the bathroom?*
- *Does each resident have individualized seating that supports him, and helps him to avoid slipping down or falling forward out of a chair?*
- *Is the dining room quiet and attractive so that eating is a relaxing and pleasant event?*
- *Does each resident have familiar furniture and mementos from home in his room?*
- *Do the sound system, radios and televisions bother the resident?*
- *Are residents who choose to go outside every day, weather permitting, able to do so?*
- *Are there quiet areas residents and families can use when they request some privacy?*

What efforts have been made to eliminate the cause? Whether the cause of the behavioral symptom is related to either physical or environmental factors, or both, efforts should be made to eliminate the cause of these symptoms. In some instances, the cause of the symptom is *not* immediately apparent. Therefore, you should work with staff to continue trying to determine the cause and to provide care without restraints.

Beulah Smith has Alzheimer's disease. She woke up every night about midnight and was very distressed for the rest of the night. Staff did an assessment of both Mrs. Smith and her environment. They talked with her family, but couldn't discover a reason for her nightly distress. Instead of restraining her in bed while further assessment continued, staff gave Mrs. Smith warm milk, and put her in a lounge chair near the nurses' desk. They covered her warmly. She would calm down and drop fitfully off to sleep. These measures worked until staff learned at a training that people with Alzheimer's disease often become very cold at night. The cause, feeling cold, was eliminated. The next night they put several extra blankets on Mrs. Smith and she slept very well.

If the cause can be found and treated or eliminated, are staff using individualized care practices? A more complete list of individualized care practices for common behavioral symptoms appears in the section following this chapter. New ways of caring continue to emerge and are used. Many of these ways are based on the good ideas of family and staff working together. Key elements are:

• *Restorative care programs*, like mobility and dining programs, help residents maintain, relearn or strengthen skills such as walking or dining.

• Use of *individualized pillows and pads* and a variety of types and sizes of chairs help to create many comfortable spots to sit for each resident. Wheelchairs are to be used primarily for transport, as they rarely offer the most comfortable place to sit.

• A *homelike environment* communicates a sense of belonging and comfort. The nursing home's sights, sounds and smells, like those at home, should be inviting. Arrangement of furniture should support socializing.

• A *physically supportive environment* features low noise, non-glare lighting, and furniture that promotes comfort and is arranged for easy sociability.

• *Supportive staff* adjust to each resident rather than each resident having to adopt to nursing home staff routines.

• Using *information about each resident's preferences* and routines, and building care around these factors, can prevent and eliminate behavioral symptoms.

What is the plan for discontinuing use of physical and/or chemical restraints? Meeting Mr. Fiske will help you understand how restraints should be time limited.

Andrew Fiske's behavior changed markedly one evening. At first, he became very agitated and dangerous to those around him. His physician and the staff could not get near him to assess the situation and find the cause of his distress. His family consented to the use of a restraint while an assessment was done. The assessment revealed that he had a urinary tract infection.

The restraint was immediately discontinued when the assessment was finished and treatment for the infection began.

Hopefully, these questions and examples have given you ideas about your role in questioning restraints. Remember always to ask questions. It's also important for you to comb through your knowledge of your relative for pieces of information that may provide clues about what the unmet need is. You might think of ways to calm your relative that the staff might not think about. Don't hesitate to speak up!

Is a Sleeping Medication a Chemical Restraint?

Sleeping medications are psychoactive drugs. Therefore, they have the potential to be used as chemical restraints. Two common situations in which this occurs involve 1) residents who get up during the night, and 2) residents who have taken a sleeping medication for many years prior to moving to a nursing home.

1) Residents who are given sleeping medications because they get up at night are being chemically restrained. The most common reasons for getting up at night are:

- need to go to the toilet
- normal, age-related changes in sleeping patterns
- staff put the residents to bed earlier than they are used to
- inability to sleep because of environmental factors, like noise or light, or untreated pain or discomfort
- sleeping too much during the day
- drinking too much caffeine.

These are all situations that can be changed, eliminating the need for a sleeping medication.

2) Many residents have taken a sleeping medication for years prior to entering a nursing home. Physicians may prescribe them after a crisis such as the death of a spouse. Sleeping medications have the potential to cause all the bad outcomes of chemical restraints, including drowsiness and incontinence. Sleeping

— *Sleeping medications have the potential to cause all the bad outcomes of chemical restraints, including drowsiness and incontinence.* —

medications also lose their effectiveness after a few months. Therefore, they should be discontinued!

There is a danger of exaggerated wakefulness when these medications are discontinued too quickly. In addition, sleeping medications should never be discontinued without:

- an agreement between staff and resident that the removal process will occur slowly
- the introduction of supportive care practices, such as back rubs, hot milk, or other individualized care measures
- the involvement of family when appropriate.

What Can You Do When Staff Insist on Using a Chemical or Physical Restraint?

You must rely on your advocacy skills when staff continue to suggest or use a physical or chemical restraint. You can ask for help solving restraint problems by:

- working with the facility to solve the problem
- getting in touch with the long-term care ombudsman
- contacting surveyors at the state's nursing home licensure agency.

Be sure to read chapter 7, "Problem Solving: Being Your Own Advocate," to learn the specifics of solving problems. This chapter also tells you about long term care ombudsmen and the licensure agency and citizen advocates. You can find out how to contact these individuals in your state by turning to Appendix 7 or via the Internet at www.nursinghomeaction.org.

A Final — Optimistic — Note on Restraints

On February 7, 1996 the American Association of Homes and Services for the Aging and the American Health Care Association — trade associations for the nursing home industry — announced a campaign to "help the nation's nursing homes end restraint use."

According to a joint press release issued by the AAHSA and AHCA, "the goal of this campaign is to decrease restraint use to zero, the next logical and ethical step in promoting high quality care."

The AAHSA and AHCA program, under the banner, *Everyone Wins!*, offers training and information for nursing home staff, families, physicians and surveyors.

If you or the staff are still insistent upon restraint use with your relative in a home, ask the administration if they are familiar with the *Everyone Wins!* program. Their own industry leaders are now advocating restraint-free care!

A complementary resource on this topic: National Citizens' Coalition for Nursing Home Reform family guides to *Avoiding Chemical Restraint Use* [and] *Avoiding Physical Restraint Use.* You will find the address in Appendix 7.

> *— All laws are subject to change. Regardless of any changes in the federal law discussed in this chapter, these standards are supported in some state laws as well as professional codes of conduct. They are good practice! They represent good care! As a family member you have every right to ask for and expect these practices for your relative. —*

Individualized Care for Common Challenges Residents Face*

RESIDENTS ARE TYPICALLY RESTRAINED DUE TO FOUR behaviors: 1) unsafe mobility/postural instability; 2) wandering; 3) agitation, confusion, and 4) interference with life support measures.

A successful restraint reduction program requires total staff support and an interdisciplinary team approach. The resident's capabilities, rather than deficits, are the focus of the care plan and treatment interventions.

Promote Resident's Function:
- Identity reason(s) for the resident's unsteadiness, need to get up, poor trunk control, etc. (For example: what medication is this person on; how much exercise has the individual been getting; is the individual hungry or thirsty; has the person been sitting too long; is the individual experiencing pain; or does the resident need to go to the bathroom?)
- Eliminate medications or combinations of medications with side effects that distort residents' balance, perceptions and/or cognitive function.
- Increase ambulation skills by giving resident opportunities to exercise. (For example: walking to and from meals or activities, developing formal exercise groups, etc.)
- Be sure residents wear comfortable well-fitting shoes or sneakers and have appropriate foot and toenail care.
- Provide supportive devices to maximize function. (For example: transfer disc, modified walkers, grab-safety bars in bathroom, elevated toilet seat, non-slip floors, etc.)
- Address residents' vision and hearing impairments.

---

*Used and adapted with permission from "Untie the Elderly," The Kendal Corporation, P.O. Box 100, Kennet Square, PA 19348

Minimize Likelihood of Residents Needing to Get Up Unaided:
- Be familiar with the residents' lifelong roles and habits to anticipate personal needs and interests, such as when they usually go to the bathroom, preferred snack times or leisure or work activities.
- Provide the resident with meaningful activity such as listening to music, assisting staff with simple tasks, or executing a repetitive task that satisfies a personal need.
- Offer residents adequate stimulation such as reading materials, talking books or an activities cart placed strategically on each unit, twenty-four hours a day.
- Vary the locations where an individual sits. Sometimes quiet areas are appreciated, but often residents want to be "where the action is."
- Explore possible alerting strategies/devices, i.e., attach call bell to resident's garment or use of portable battery-operated alarms that monitor the individual's movements.

Customize Seating for Individual Postural Needs:
- Provide flexion at hips and knees and lateral support with wedge cushions, positioning pillows, and/or deep inclined seats to minimize slumping, falling to the side or sliding out of chair.
- Ensure that the most comfortable seating is available and that the resident is not expected to sit for prolonged periods. Offer a variety of sitting arrangements, such as Lay-Z-Boys, Barc-a-loungers, rockers, deep-seated high-backed chairs, or soft comfortable wing chairs.
- Prevent tipping of wheelchairs with anti-tipping devices which are commercially available.
- Wheelchairs are for transportation only. If a resident is unable to propel the wheelchair independently, he/she should be seated in it solely for transportation purposes.

Ensure a Safe Environment for Resident:
- Monitor environment for safety hazards.
- Modify environment with optimal lighting in residents' rooms and bathrooms, appropriately placed safety bars, removal of wheels from overbed table and other furniture (the resident may lean on for support).

- Keep beds as low to the floor as possible. (Low beds are commercially available.)
- Ongoing resident evaluation and monitoring for bed safety. (Contact Kendall Corp., see footnote on page 91 for pamphlet "A Guide to Bed Safety Bed Rails in Hospitals, Nursing Homes and Home Health Care.")

Make Environment as Home-Like as Possible:
- Encourage residents to surround themselves with personal furniture and possessions. This helps in recognition of one's room and provides a comfortable, secure haven in an often strange environment.
- Encourage nursing staff to wear ordinary clothing rather than uniforms.
- Eliminate, or at least reduce, the use of a public address system. Voices coming over these systems are stressful and confusing for frail residents.

Decrease the Risks Associated with Resident Wandering:
- Provide opportunities for the resident to have a sense of purpose.
- Schedule activities that are consistent with the resident's interest and cognitive ability.
- Offer opportunities for the resident to phone, listen to tapes or view videos of persons(s) he/she wants to find.
- Provide companionship and one-on-one attention. Identify the emotional needs the resident is trying to meet by wandering. Listen to and validate each resident's feelings.
- Enlist *all* staff to do their part in keeping track of a wandering resident. *It's not just a nursing responsibility*. Make it a shared responsibility of all departments by assigning one staff member to supervise a wanderer for short periods of time.
- Provide comfortable rocking chairs to offer relaxation and satisfy the need for constant motion.
- Give the resident opportunities to exercise.
- Modify the environment to discourage people from wandering into inappropriate areas and/or exiting facility:
  - Create a grid with masking tape on floor in front of doorway.
  - Put mirror on door.
  - Camouflage the door with wallpaper, window treatment, etc.

- Install alarm system.
- Attach an 18-inch wide barrier strip across the doorway with velcro.
- Put dark mat or felt circle on floor in front of doors.
- Place stop sign on door.

Accept the Fact that Restless, Anxious Residents Need to Walk When Able:

- Make environment as safe as possible and promote freedom to wander.
- Place resident's name and picture on door of his/her room (preferably a photo taken 20-30 years earlier).
- Learn the resident's daily routines and patterns of movement. Provide activity that makes use of the wandering "agenda behavior." For example, encourage resident to assist staff in simple tasks such as folding napkins, setting table, decorating bulletin board, sorting papers, dusting, pushing laundry cart, etc.
- Install a curtained swinging cafe door with a buzzer on the entrance of the resident's room. (Serves to alert staff of resident's movement, especially at night.)
- Provide a safe enclosed area outside with a walking path and shaded benches for rest stops.

Educate Staff in Techniques of Assessing and Caring for Residents Who are Agitated:

- Seek underlying causes for behavior. (Ask the person what is the matter; check medications; is individual experiencing discomfort?)
- Use a calm approach when addressing a resident. Be gentle and consistent.
- Increase communication with a resident.
- Be familiar with the clinical stages of dementia to ensure that activity programs are appropriate for each resident's cognitive ability.
- Engage resident in structured activity that provides meaningful activity throughout day, i.e., OT, PT, recreation, special sessions for special needs, etc.
- Have the resident listen to relaxation tapes.

- Respect a resident's need for personal space. "Back off" from resident who is acting in an aggressive manner until he/she feels calmer.
- Provide for a consistent caregiver to ensure continuity of care. This will decrease the likelihood of agitated behavior and increase sensitivity to the individual's needs.

Re-Evaluate Life Support Measures:
- Consider wisdom and ethics of approach.
- Encourage residents to make a living will or durable power of attorney for health care while they are competent.
- Explore with physicians the residents' right to dignity, comfort and autonomy.
- Discuss residents' rights with family members. Talk about what the resident wants.
- Evaluate the need for feeding tube; consider alternatives such as hydration by mouth.
- Evaluate the need for urinary catheters; allow incontinence or attempt a rigorous bladder training program.
- Remove tubes which appear to be causing resident major distress.
- Consider insertion of tube directly into stomach instead of naso-gastric tubes.
- Cover IV tubing with long sleeves.
- Disguise gastrostomy tube with flextone binders over abdomen.
- Fit stockinette over small nurf ball held in hand or partially inflated to air splint over elbow to prevent resident from pulling naso-gastric tube as a *temporary* measure.

Nurture Positive Staff-Resident-Family Relationships:
- Provide primary nursing care — avoid rotation of caregivers.
- Maintain communications with family members. Family input is invaluable in understanding resident behavior and developing appropriate care plans.
- Understand each resident as an individual with personal needs and desires. Care plans must be individualized and flexible to meet the ever-changing status of the resident.

Chapter 6

Advocating for Quality of Life

- **Step Up**—and pay attention to things that make a day good.

  - **Speak Up**—about important choices and daily routines.

    - **Advocate for Good Care**—and residents and staff "win".

As you visit with Aunt Dora in a nursing home, she's irritable and looks tired. After you've talked for a while, she tells you what's bothering her. Every morning she's awakened by a nurse assistant, who enters the room, opens the blinds, and chirps, "Good morning, it's time to get you dressed and down to the dining room!" Dora is helped with her clothes and whisked down to breakfast — ready or not. Not surprisingly, your aunt begins every day feeling out of sorts. Before she moved into the home, Aunt Dora always liked to awaken slowly, taking time to stretch and ease into the day. She never was very talkative first thing in the morning, she liked to be up and moving a while before eating...

Think about your own day...
Is your mood affected by:
- getting a good night's sleep?
- waking up quietly and gradually?
- having hot coffee in the morning?
- listening to your style of music?
- hearing constant, often loud, noise?
- deciding when to eat?
- choosing what to wear?
- seeing dust balls on the floor?
- turning lights on and off as you like?
- being able to say "No" when you don't want something?
- having privacy when you need it?

- living in cluttered surroundings?
- feeling safe and secure in your home?
- receiving a friendly response from others?
- deciding what you do and when you do it?
- having some control over what is in your room and how it is arranged?

The list could go on and on. You're probably aware of a number of things that influence the quality of your life every day. Things that leave you with a feeling of having had a good day.

What happens if you miss several of the items on your quality list? Do you become irritable, impatient, unsettled, restless, or anxious? What does it take to restore your sense of self and your positive attitude? If you're like most people, it takes returning to your typical routines, having your choices respected and your needs met.

Now that she's in an institution, will Aunt Dora have to give up those needs and conform to the home's way of starting her day?

No! In a radical departure from the old way of doing things, nursing homes are now expected to adapt to each resident! The "Quality of Life" section of the Nursing Home Reform law set new standards for individualization of care. Most homes are conforming with these standards to some degree. They're providing care tailored to individual needs and desires. (You've read about them in chapter 2 on residents' rights and chapter 3 on assessment and care planning. Remember Mr. Zentoff's assessment and care planning!) You can use these standards to help the nursing home support Aunt Dora's customary life patterns. But isn't it unrealistic to expect a nursing home to support an individually defined "quality of life" for each resident? What's the bottom line here?

What is Quality of Life in a Nursing Home?

"Quality of life" sounds like a very broad concept. And it is, yet you've just identified several factors that significantly influence the quality of *your* daily life. Everyone can name key factors that contribute to the quality of their lives. Quality of life is heavily shaped for all of us by the myriad tangible acts that make up our days and the nature of our interactions with others.

And it's just that simple to focus on the meaning of "quality of life" in a nursing home. According to survey research, residents feel good about living in a home if they have *kind, caring staff,* have *choices and control over their daily lives*, and are able to *maintain their normal routines.**

Your Relative's Perspective
To begin considering your own relative's present quality of life, it helps to start by thinking about her routines prior to entering a nursing home.
- What gave meaning to her life?
- What were sources of pride?
- How did she organize her day?

Then think about how many of these elements are present in her daily life in the nursing home. Talk with your relative about the essence of her daily life now. Ask her:
- What adds to the enjoyment of each day?
- What detracts from it?

If your relative can't tell you this information, use your knowledge of her past to think about how she would answer if she could. Also consider her behavior. Does it give any clues about her response to these questions?

A sample list of personal information you or your relative could give nursing home staff to help them individualize your relative's care is in Appendix 4.

What Is the Basic Standard for Quality of Life?
As we have seen, the law features quality of life as one of its main tenets. Here is the text:

A nursing facility must care for its residents in such a manner and in such an environment as will promote maintenance or enhancement of the quality of life of each resident.

The standard was set by the Nursing Home Reform Law. Homes that understand quality of life know that quality of life and quality of care are intertwined. You learned this in the previous chapter on restraint-free care. Care must be delivered in a way that supports quality of life.

— *Care must be delivered in a way that supports quality of life.* —

---

*A Consumer Perspective on Quality Care: The Residents' Point of View. 1985. National Citizens' Coalition for Nursing Home Reform, 1424 16th St., NW, Washington, DC 20036, www.nursinghomeaction.org.

Each individual resident's quality of life should be maintained or improved by the way the facility delivers care and the way the environment supports the person. Quality of life should not decline for an individual just because he now lives in a nursing home.

Just as the quality of *care* standard means that residents shouldn't develop certain *physical* conditions after they enter a facility, the quality of *life* standard is that residents' emotional well-being also should not worsen.

What's more, quality of life is to be *individualized*. The central components of quality of life for one resident may not be the same for another resident. Facilities cannot rely on a few standard approaches to maintaining and enhancing quality of life for all residents.

Group and individual activities that are of interest to residents are vital to the quality of life in a home. Activities are to be individualized for residents by the activities staff just as care routines are to be designed for each resident. An environment conducive to informal conversations, where residents are freely sitting together, talking or working on common projects is supportive of friendships and the quality of life.

You might be thinking, "This all sounds great, but how can I make it happen for my relative? Is the facility going to listen to me when I suggest changes to improve *her* quality of life?"

Let's take another look at Aunt Dora.

How Does Quality of Life Become a Reality?

Residents' Rights. *When you locate and re-read the information on "residents' rights" provided by Aunt Dora's facility, you note several items that lead you to believe that Aunt Dora does not have to change her routines to match the facility's schedule. For example, you read that:*

- "residents can choose activities, schedules, and health care consistent with their interests, assessments and plans of care;"
- "residents can make choices about aspects of life in the facility that are significant to each resident."

This is only the beginning! Reading these rights is a real boost — you know you're on the right track. It's OK for Aunt Dora to expect a morning routine that is consistent with her customary patterns.

Assessment. *You tell Aunt Dora what you've learned and ask how she would like her morning to go. What she tells you confirms your* *memories of her lifelong routine. It's no wonder that she is irritable and tired with a morning routine that is so opposite to her natural patterns!*

As the two of you talk, Aunt Dora says, "I told them how I want to begin my day when I moved here!" You vaguely recall staff asking lots of questions and mentioning an "assessment." Maybe there was something about customary routines. Someone in the facility does have this type of information about Aunt Dora's routines and preferences, but what do you do next?

Care Planning. *Looking back at the list of residents' rights, you see the right to participate in planning care and treatment. That's it! The care plan meeting was a time when staff talked with Aunt Dora and you about what they would be doing. They noted that Aunt Dora likes showers instead of tub baths.*

You go to Aunt Dora's nurse and ask for a review of the care plan to see what adjustments can be made in your aunt's morning routine. Aunt Dora and you meet with the charge nurse, your aunt's morning nurse assistant, and the dietary supervisor. Your aunt describes the routine she prefers, with you present for moral support.

Everyone agrees that your aunt can awaken on her own. She'll use the call light when she's ready for assistance with dressing, and will let the nurse assistant know when she's ready for breakfast. Your aunt probably will be at the second seating for breakfast each day. Should she miss the official breakfast time, cereal, fruit and some toast will be available on her unit when she's ready.

As you drive home after this meeting, you realize that residents' rights, assessment, and care planning all work together to make a significant difference in Aunt Dora's quality of life. Each one of these helps the nursing home know Aunt Dora as an individual. Residents' rights also entitle your aunt to speak out and make choices about her daily life. You're feeling good about helping Aunt Dora begin each day the way she has for years — the way she wants to!

Are there Other Standards that Support Quality of Life?

Yes! In the preceding example you saw how Aunt Dora's quality of life was improved by drawing upon other standards of care and practice. These were initially set forth in the law. Now they are commonly accepted. These will be briefly highlighted so you'll have them in one place as a reference when quality of life questions arise. You can think of these other sections as *tools* to help facilities support each resident's quality of life. They are also your tools when specific quality of life issues need to be addressed.

Residents' Rights. This main subsection of the law is not just about legal requirements or entitlement. The law clearly identifies residents' rights as major ingredients of quality of life. (You'll recall our detailed discussion of residents' rights in chapter 2. A complete list of residents' federal rights can be found in Appendix 3.)

Residents' rights are like highway signs: they give directions. If residents are supported and encouraged to fully exercise all of their rights, the facility will meet the quality of life requirements. *Residents' rights give meaning to the term "quality of life."*

In the beginning of this chapter, you identified factors that influence your daily quality of life. At the root of many of your factors was your ability to be in control and to make choices. Would you believe *control* and *choice* are the root of many of the residents' rights? They are!

If facilities are upholding residents' rights, they'll be helping residents achieve quality of life. Facilities which are fully implementing residents' rights are responsive to resident

- choice
- communication with staff
- participation in planning their own care and in the life of the facility and the community, and
- decision-making.

Resident Assessment. The required assessment process guides facility staff in gathering specific information about each resident's abilities, relationships, and patterns. This procedure is an opportunity for you to help the facility support or enhance quality of life for your relative. To get the most out of this process, both you and your relative should participate. The nursing home staff need to learn as much as possible about your

— This procedure is an opportunity for you to help the facility support or enhance quality of life for your relative. —

relative's usual routines and preferences. In other words, they need to know what impacts the *quality* of the resident's daily life — the things that comfort as well as annoy your relative. They need a list with similar types of factors as those you identified at the beginning of this chapter.

A section on the standard assessment form called "Customary Routines" guides the staff in asking for this kind of information. The social worker, dietician, activities professional, or nurse may ask additional questions about the resident's preferences and patterns. Don't hesitate to offer more information than is requested about what is important to your relative's daily life.

As much as possible, the resident should be the one who provides this information. In some cases, you may need to supplement the information or discuss it with staff. Either way, thinking through the details beforehand will help you prepare. Organize the information in such a way that staff can access it easily: that is, *write it so your audience — the staff — can and will read it!* Remember they have a big job. (Chapter 3 has more information on resident assessment.)

Care Planning. As we discussed in chapter 3, the care planning meeting is an important tool. Care planning is a key time to talk about making the nursing home environment more conducive to your relative's comfort and enjoyment of life. To get the most from these opportunities, prepare carefully in advance.

Before the meeting, encourage your friend or relative to think about quality of life factors that make a difference each day. List areas that need to be changed.

...Is care *delivered in a way* that supports, or improves, the resident's enjoyment of everyday life?

...Is the nursing home *environment* supportive of quality of life?

...If the answer to either of those questions is "no," what needs to be changed?

...What are some possible solutions that will bring about these changes and improve your relative's quality of life?

After thinking through these kinds of questions, you and your relative will be better prepared to discuss problems and solutions in a care planning meeting. If there are situations that need to be handled before the next scheduled care planning meeting, you can request a meeting to review the resident's care. Like resident assessment, a more detailed discussion of the care planning process also appears in chapter 3.

Survey Process. There is yet another valuable tool to use in focusing on quality of life. Each nursing home is *surveyed* to determine if it is complying with the law and regulations.

(To learn more about the survey process, turn to chapter 7, "Problem Solving.")

One big part of the survey process looks at quality of life *through the eyes of residents*. Surveyors interview individual residents, a group of residents, and some family members. In addition, anyone who wishes may request a time to speak with the survey team. You or your relative can ask to talk with the survey team if there is something you want them to know.

The purpose of these interviews is to find out about the residents' view of quality of life in the facility. Surveyors may ask residents such questions as:

...Is there anything that would make this facility more comfortable for you?

...Are you served foods that you like to eat?

...Is there some activity that you would like to do that is not available here?

...How does the facility respond when you make recommendations about your care and life?

In addition to conducting interviews, surveyors must observe *environmental* factors pertinent to quality of life. Surveyors are directed to consider questions such as these:

...Are residents' rooms, toilets and bath facilities, along with common areas like corridors and dining halls, comfortable and homelike from the residents' perspective?

...Are sounds at a comfortable level during evenings and at nighttime?

...Do environmental adaptations *enhance* residents' independence, self-control, and well-being?

The survey process underscores the importance of quality of life. You might ask your "Aunt Dora" these survey questions to see whether there is something that needs to be discussed in a care planning meeting, or perhaps brought to the attention of a survey team.

Quality of life, from the survey standpoint, does capture the many "little things" that give meaning to each of us daily. The questions surveyors ask reflect *choice, communication, participation and decision-making* — everyday hallmarks of quality.

What Would You Do?

Check your understanding of quality of life and of ways to use the tools listed above, by reading the scenarios that follow. Read the *Situation,* then test yourself by thinking through the steps you would take. Then read the *Response* to see if it is similar to your ideas. There may be several approaches which would result in the desired change, so don't be hard on yourself if your solution differs from that of the *Response* as we've described it.

Situation #1. *Your mother always made the transition from a hectic day to a relaxing evening with a cup of hot decaffeinated coffee. She complains about missing this ritual in the nursing home and of having difficulty unwinding for the evening. When she asked the kitchen staff for coffee they spoke to her like she was a child trying to break the rules. Their response was so harsh that she opted against talking to the dietary supervisor. Your mother resigns herself to thinking it's better to put up with things the way staff want them to be.*
What would you do?
Response #1. *You persuade her to accompany you to talk with the dietary supervisor because you know how important a role the evening coffee played in your mother's daily patterns. After some discussion, the dietary supervisor agrees that your mother can have decaffeinated coffee in the evenings. Everyone helps plan when and where it will be available. A few days later, your mother reports feeling more at home and finding it easier to relax and sleep after resuming this soothing routine.*

Situation #2. *Your uncle grew up at a time when it wasn't customary to take a bath every day. Now that he's in a nursing facility, he feels the staff is bullying him into taking too many baths. He is resentful and staff tell you he is pushing them away. No one wants to bathe him because his resistance puts them behind schedule. Then they get in trouble with the nurse. You see your uncle is becoming hostile and withdrawn.*
One morning you arrive just as a nurse assistant is trying to get your uncle to bathe. You hear her telling him how bad he smells and that no one wants to be around him because of his body odor. You realize that the nursing home has assaulted your uncle's dignity, self-esteem, and well-being because he's simply trying to preserve his familiar pattern of weekly baths.
What would you do?
Response #2. *You enter the room as the nurse assistant leaves. After talking with your uncle, you ask the charge nurse to sit down with the*

two of you to review your uncle's care plan. The three of you discuss the importance of basic hygiene and various ways to meet this need. You also talk about the way staff approach your uncle and his right to dignity. Your uncle agrees to bathe in the whirlpool twice a week, with spot bathing at other times. It becomes obvious that if staff adjust to your uncle's routine, respecting his choices in bathing, keeping him clean will not take extra time and energy. The nurse agrees to talk with the nurse assistant about how to respond to residents, especially when they choose a different routine. She also promises to assign the nurse assistant who best understands your uncle to help him with hygiene needs.

Quality of Life IS Possible

At the heart of quality of life for each of us is the need to be treated with kindness and dignity, and to be able to exercise control and choice in daily life decisions.

There's no magic to meeting these needs in a nursing home. It is attainable! Maintaining or enhancing a resident's quality of life takes:

- *knowledge* of the factors that influence the individual's quality of life and
- *creativity* and *flexibility* to ensure these factors exist to the greatest extent possible in the nursing home.

It's a two-step process that can make an enormous difference in how a resident regards life in her new home.

If you're wondering what to do if a problem arises without an easy solution, keep reading! The next chapter, "Problem Solving: Being Your Own Advocate," is full of useful tips on how to approach facility staff. It also discusses problem-solving techniques and other resources to help you if the facility is uncooperative.

— All laws are subject to change. Regardless of any changes in the federal law discussed in this chapter, these standards are supported in some state laws as well as professional codes of conduct. They are good practice! They represent good care! As a family member you have every right to ask for and expect these practices for your relative. —

Chapter 7

Problem Solving:
Being Your Own Advocate

- **Step Up** — Know the nursing home complaint process.

  - **Speak Up** — Use effective problem solving skills.

    - **Advocate For Good Care** — Locate help outside the nursing home when necessary.

June Myers dropped in at the Rocking River Care Center after a harried day teaching seventh-grade English. Fortunately, the facility was close to her school, so she could stop often on her way home to see her mother, Theresa Miller, who had been in the home for more than six months due to a stroke. June had begun to dread the visits. Driving the last few blocks she wondered what she would find this time, and how she could deal with seeing her mother lying in a wet bed again. She just couldn't stand knowing how humiliated and embarrassed her mother was in this condition.

When June walked in her mother's room, Mrs. Miller turned her head away and began to cry softly. "I put my light on," she whispered. "I tried to call and tell them I had to go to the bathroom. No one came. I'm so miserable."

June felt her blood pressure rising. This was it. She stormed down the hall, grabbed the first aide she saw, and shouted angrily at her, loud enough to be heard at the nurse's station at the other end of the hall. "Why can't you take care of my mother? Isn't that what all that money I pay is supposed to be for?" she screamed. "How many more times must I come in here and find her wet and dirty?"

Rushing to the scene, a nurse pleaded with June to lower her voice. "I don't care how many people I disturb," she boomed. "Don't you think my mother is disturbed when she can't get anyone to answer the call light?"

The nurse told June that one of the aides was just going into her mother's room. She also informed her that two aides had called in sick that day, and no one could be found to replace them.

"Well that's not my problem," June snapped. "My problem is my mother and I'm sick and tired of all your excuses." With that, she retreated into her mother's room and slammed the door.

Well, Now We Know What Not to Do!

June was understandably frustrated, and most people would agree that she has not solved the problem. Moreover, she has unintentionally created a lot of ill will for herself and perhaps for her mother.

— Knowing when and how to confront problems will help both you and other friends and family members to get them resolved. —

Basic problem-solving skills are an essential part of all relationships. They are particularly important when you are responsible for someone else's care. Knowing when and how to confront problems will help both you and other friends and family members to get them resolved. Consider some of the things that went wrong in June's confrontation. She:

- stored up problems
- tried to approach the problem without waiting until she cooled down
- put staff on the defensive
- didn't consult her mother to see how she would prefer to handle the situation
- laid blame rather than stated the problem.

If you look back to a time when things went wrong after a long and hectic day, you can probably identify with June and her desire to lash out. Obviously, a lot of things were going wrong with her mother's care at this facility.

What's Going On Here?

Most people know how problem situations occur in their daily lives, at work, and at home. When we think about the number of people living and working together in a nursing home, it does seem inevitable that problems will arise.

They arise because of understaffing or poor management at the facility. They also stem from residents' illnesses, dependencies or mental confusion. The problems often are linked to lack of information or differing expectations. Frequent complaints involve quality of food and loss of personal possessions. Problems commonly stem from unanswered call bells, conflicts with roommates, and inadequate attention to personal hygiene.

You are fortunate if you are dealing with a nursing home whose administrator has an "open-door policy," where concerns are welcomed, staff listen to residents and families, and problems are quickly resolved.

Unfortunately, this is not always the case. Sometimes, facility staff avoid problems. Or, when problems are brought to their attention, staff may say they don't get paid enough, can't find enough trained staff, or that nurse assistants don't show up for work.

For staff who truly are committed to quality care, working in a nursing home is among the most trying challenges the human services field has to offer. Time and money always seem in demand. Thus, even good advocacy often encounters defensive attitudes. But when family members approach problem-solving with anger and accusations, they run the risk of sacrificing a fair hearing for their concerns.

Just as you must be a strong advocate and speak forcefully on the resident's behalf, you must act thoughtfully to ensure best results. The next section offers some skills and resources to help you strike that balance.

Informal Problem Solving: Important Things to Consider

You encounter a problem with your family member's care. To whom do you go? How do you get it resolved? Here are some things to consider.

• **Do you know how the administrator wants residents and families to deal with concerns?** Some administrators may want you to talk directly to the department head who is involved with the complaint, such as the food services supervisor for diet issues, the director of nursing for care issues, or the activity director or social worker if the problem involves the areas they oversee. Other administrators may choose to have all problems brought directly to them. Is there a grievance process that the facility uses? Should

— The better you know how the system works, the better your chances of success. —

you put these things in writing? The better you know how the system works, the better your chances of success.

• **Have you let complaints accumulate until you are so frustrated that you will be unable to state your concerns objectively?** Better to take them one at a time, when you can be calmer and less angry in your initial approach.

• **What is the specific complaint?** Just saying that the food is terrible and the care is awful makes it difficult for the staff to know what you want and where to start to correct the problem. In contrast, stating clearly that the facility has not followed the low-salt diet your mother's doctor ordered for her lets the staff know what they need to do. The more specific you can be, the greater the possibility the problem can be corrected. If necessary, keep records of what happened and when it occurred.

• **Whose problem is it?** If your mother's clothes aren't color coordinated, does she care? It is important to ask yourself this question and try to decide whether this is a critical issue to address, or if you can overlook this matter and focus your concerns on larger issues.

• **Can you prioritize the issues?** In the example above, the clothing issue may be much less important than the fact that she is only getting a bath once week. Are there minor annoyances, which do not overly concern your mother, that you can disregard in order to turn your attention toward resolving more significant problems?

• **How does the resident want to approach the problem?** Does she simply need to air feelings rather than have you confront staff about a problem? Sometimes, just listening can be the most effective thing you can do. The resident has to live in the nursing home twenty-four hours a day. The resident's wishes must be respected. This doesn't mean, though, that you shouldn't encourage problem-solving.

— The resident has to live in the nursing home twenty-four hours a day. The resident's wishes must be respected. —

Going Up the Ladder

Imagine that you have considered all these matters. The problem is that your father must have his food cut up into small pieces at meal time in order for him to be able to handle it. He has frequently left his dinner half-eaten because he did not receive help. You have spoken to the aides in the dining room and they have assured you they will take care of the problem. But still it goes on. After contacting the food-service supervisor, things improved for about a week, then the problem returned. Already exasperated, you become alarmed when you notice your father looks as if he's losing weight. It is time to go up the ladder.

Requesting a Meeting: A Few Good Tips

In the above example, the problem has grown to include not simply the food service but the fact that your concerns and repeated efforts to report the problem haven't fixed it. One possibility is to request an appointment with the administrator so that you can work out a solution. This may take place in the context of a care-planning conference, as described in chapter 3, or simply during a special meeting on this particular issue, as discussed below. A care conference or problem-solving meeting should include all those who have responsibility for resolving the problem, along with everyone else concerned about how the problem affects the resident's well-being.

What you should avoid doing is simply catching the administrator in the hall on his way to a meeting and expecting to have his full attention.

Before the Meeting...

In preparation for a meeting to discuss a problem, it is important to think about the **result you are seeking.** In addition, you should take some time to consider the following questions.

• **Are there other people with the same concerns?** You may not be able to speak for other families, but if you are having a problem, others likely have similar concerns. If the issue involves food or dining problems, the resident council (described in next section) may have discussed the problem in the past.

• **Have you personally observed the problem?** Have you recorded the times and dates when it occurred? Have you recorded the attempts you have made to get the problem solved? Times, dates and person you spoke to? Can you state the problem objectively, focusing on the effect and outcome for the resident? Simply talking about what "they" did or didn't do will only put staff on the defensive.

• **Are you familiar with the regulations or residents' rights that may apply to this problem?** Look back over the chapters in this book to see whether any rights in federal and state laws or regulations relate to this situation. Prior to the meeting, you may wish to speak to the ombudsman, who may help you find the appropriate regulation. While it's not necessary to quote specific laws and regulations, it is helpful to demonstrate your knowledge of the pertinent regulations.

• **Will the people who can solve the problem be at the conference?** Try to ensure that the individuals who are in a position to solve the problem will be present, and that enough time has been allotted to sufficiently discuss the problem.

During the Meeting...

Establish a sense of cooperation and inclusion. Assume that staff do value satisfied customers and thus will want to know about, and fix, the problem.

• **Hear staff out, but don't lose sight of your goal: the resident's well-being.** Even with your best communication style, staff are likely to put up their guard. The administrator may blame aides who call in sick, regulations that entail too much time-consuming paperwork,

> *— Hear staff out, but don't lose sight of your goal: the resident's well-being. —*

or reimbursement rates that are too low. Remember: these circumstances are their management problem, not yours. Your role is to advocate for good care for the resident.

• **Offer solutions about the problem's cause and its solution.** If your family member has a particularly agitated reaction to an event, explore what may have caused the response. Ask staff whether they have tried to anticipate what provokes these symptoms. For example, people with diminished mental capacity often refuse to shower because they greatly fear what, to them, seems like an unknown and dangerous experience.

• **Don't leave the meeting without a clear understanding of what you can expect.** Know what you should do if the problem continues. Also be confident that staff know how you would like the problem handled. It's a particularly good idea to follow up the meeting with a note of thanks, reviewing the problem and summarizing how the nursing home has agreed to handle it.

How to Submit a Complaint

There are several organizations — identified in the next section of this chapter — that are equipped to help with complaints about the quality of care in a nursing home. Most will take your complaint by phone, but it is preferable to put it in writing. To submit a complaint:

• Be as specific as possible regarding your concerns. See if you can answer the *who, what, where, when,* and *why* questions in your letter to them. The timing of their response is usually based on the severity of the complaint.

• Include any relevant documents and the names of other persons who may be contacted.

• State that you would like a copy of the report sent to you.

Where to Turn: Important Support Systems for Advocates
Inside the Nursing Home
Resident and Family Councils. Many nursing homes have active *resident councils,* made up of residents and representatives, which gather regularly and may make recommendations concerning the facility's policies. A council can provide a strong, unified voice for residents' concerns and opinions about their living conditions. For certain problems, such as those relating to food and meal service, the resident council can prove particularly effective.

Most nursing homes have organized some type of *family or community council.* Depending on their structure and format, these groups can provide effective forums for discussing and following through on concerns that affect many residents in the facility. Some family groups mainly provide support and information; others actively advocate for changes in care. While regular attendance at these group meetings may be difficult for people with other family, work and community obligations, it is important for advocates to be part of this group. Try to schedule your regular visits around these meetings.

— *Nationwide, family councils are helping to change the way nursing homes care for residents.* —

Nationwide, family councils are helping to change the way nursing homes care for residents. If your facility does not have an active family council, look into organizing one.

In one recent example, a family group, unable to get their problem solved with the facility, contacted the facility's corporate office. After a series of meetings, the administrator was dismissed and the families were asked to be involved in the hiring process for a new administrator.

Outside the Nursing Home

Your mother has gone into the nursing home with a broken hip. Before her Medicare benefits ran out, she received physical therapy. Now that she is on Medicaid, the doctor has ordered that she receive assistance walking three times a day. But she is not getting the rehabilitation as ordered. You've met with the facility staff and the problem has not been resolved. It is time to call for additional help. It is time to talk with someone who may have the authority or ability to correct the problem.

The Ombudsman Program. The ombudsman is a consumer advocate responsible for investigating and attempting to resolve complaints made by, or on behalf of, residents of long-term care facilities. In most parts of the country, there is an ombudsman assigned to every nursing home.

Start by identifying the ombudsman for your facility. Usually, there will be a sign with the ombudsman's name and phone number posted in the facility. If you can't locate it, ask the nursing home's director of social services for the information. Or,

— Start by identifying the ombudsman for your facility. —

contact your State Long-Term Care Ombudsman. (A list of each State Long-Term Care Ombudsman appears in Appendix 7.) The state ombudsman will identify the right person to contact.

Once you have located the facility's ombudsman, explain the problem, telling her who you have contacted and what you have done. Ask for advice. She will probably know if there have been similar complaints from other residents. The ombudsman will consider your information confidential, unless you and the resident give her permission to speak to others on the resident's behalf. The ombudsman will want to talk to the resident personally and conduct a separate investigation of her own. When this is completed, the ombudsman will work with you and the resident to develop the best course of action.

In the case of the resident with the broken hip, the ombudsman may wish to find out whether the resident's physician knows that rehabilitation is not occurring as ordered. She may also suggest calling another meeting with the ombudsman present or making a complaint to the licensing agency, as described in the next section of this chapter.

While the ombudsman program attempts to solve problems at their origin — within the facility — the program depends on regulatory agencies to step in when necessary. The ombudsman program and most regulatory agencies will, on the request of a resident or family member, attempt to solve a problem without identifying the resident. For example, in a case where the problem is widespread, such as cold food, it is easy to protect the resident's identity. But in a case relating to an individual problem, it is often impossible to avoid disclosing the resident's name. *It is important to remember that any form of retaliation against a resident who brought a complaint is illegal.* (Which is not to suggest that it can't happen.)

State Licensing and Certification Offices. Federal and state governments regulate nursing home care. The federal government establishes standards of care for nursing homes to meet in order to receive Medicaid and Medicare payments. State governments work in partnership with federal Medicaid programs and oversee nursing home care through their role as protectors of the public interest.

The licensing and certification office is generally housed in the state health department. This office is responsible for handling complaints. It also inspects nursing homes on a regular basis to ensure they meet standards. Yearly surveys identify deficiencies in areas like residents' rights, quality of life, quality of care, activities, social services, environment, safety. If deficiencies are found, the facility is responsible for correcting them. Licensing and certification officials can take numerous enforcement actions to sanction facilities that do not meet standards. These include a ban on admissions, civil fines or close monitoring.

Residents and families are currently an important part of the survey process. During each annual survey, a sample of residents is interviewed extensively, along with a few family members. In addition, surveyors meet with the resident council to learn how well the nursing home is meeting residents' needs. Residents and family members are urged to speak with surveyors even though they may not have been individually selected for interviews.

A copy of the survey and plan of correction must be available in the facility. It also can be obtained at the licensing and certification office and, in most cases, through the Ombudsman Program.

Regulatory Agencies. If your concern involves the action of the administrator, a nurse, a physician, a therapist, or a nurse assistant, you may wish to make a report to the board which licenses or certifies that individual. You can get information regarding the procedures or addresses from your local or state Ombudsman Program.

Resources for Reporting Neglect or Abuse. The definition of abuse generally covers a broad range of actions and practices involving the infliction of physical or mental injury: striking, slapping, shoving, shaking, menacing, harassing, inappropriate use of restraints, nonconsensual sexual conduct. Financial exploitation and neglect are other forms of abuse. State laws vary as to how, and where, abuse must be reported.

Several agencies have responsibility for responding to complaints involving this type of serious misconduct — especially conduct that results in injury. For example, each state designates a particular agency (usually within the department of health) to receive complaints about abuse committed by certified nurse assistants. State agencies that license nursing home administrators, physicians and other professionals receive abuse-related complaints involving those individuals.

In most states, the local department of social services is responsible for investigating abuse complaints. Law enforcement officials are often called upon to investigate.

It is crucial that abuse in nursing homes never go unrecognized or unreported. The ombudsman can provide help in knowing whom to call.

Litigation. If repeated attempts to resolve a problem have failed, or if there has been serious abuse or neglect, taking the situation to an attorney may be an appropriate course of action. Seek an attorney experienced in personal injury and civil trial law who is familiar with nursing home issues. Keep in mind, however, that litigation is costly and usually very slow.

Citizen Advocacy Groups. In many states or local communities there are citizen groups made up of advocates who are seeking advocacy improvements in nursing home care. They may be able to assist with individual problems or systemic issues. The National Citizens' Coalition for Nursing Home Reform (NCCNHR) can assist in providing information about these groups. See Appendix 7, for contact information.

The National Citizens' Coalition for Nursing Home Reform. Based in Washington, D.C., NCCNHR's members include consumer groups, local and state ombudsman programs, and individual citizen advocates across the country. Since the 1970s, NCCNHR has worked to improve the quality of care and quality of life in nursing homes and other long-term care facilities.

NCCNHR led the movement for passage of the 1987 Nursing Home Reform Law. The law established new standards in care — standards which are now accepted practice by many professionals and support staff in nursing homes. Today, NCCNHR continues to work with state and federal lawmakers, policy experts and regulatory officials, monitoring laws and regulations to ensure they promote residents' rights and well-being.

— NCCNHR continues to work with state and federal lawmakers, policy experts and regulatory officials, monitoring laws and regulations and ensuring that they promote residents' rights and well-being. —

NCCNHR's information clearinghouse offers numerous publications on special areas of concern, like restraint reduction and effective care planning, as well as information on nursing home law and regulations. NCCNHR responds to thousands of clearinghouse requests annually, offering information, ideas and referrals. NCCNHR also provides consultation, training, and community education on a range of long-term care issues.

Each fall, NCCNHR brings together advocates, including family members like yourself, from around the country to discuss and learn more about current issues affecting the quality of care and quality of life of nursing home residents during a four-day annual meeting. In 1993, NCCNHR was designated the National Long-Term Care Ombudsman Resource Center under a federal grant from the Administration on Aging. See Appendix 7, page 149, for information on how to contact NCCNHR.

Common Factors for Quality Nursing Homes

This book is not about how to choose a "good" nursing home, but it is helpful to recognize the kinds of things that the home's residents, and the community it serves, value. By identifying the positive aspects of a home, we may be better able to understand why problems arise and how to avoid them.

Most people involved in the nursing home field — caregivers and advocates alike — agree there are certain factors common to quality nursing homes. They include:

- consistent and responsive ownership
- stable, well-trained staff
- community interaction
- a philosophy of resident-directed care
- a mission to eliminate restraints
- teamwork between management and staff
- respect and advocacy for residents' rights.

In nursing homes where care is poor, these features are often lacking. Many facilities are owned by large, out-of-state corporations whose primary responsibility may be a good return for investors. Advocates who raise concerns about poor care often are told that nursing home care is costly and that it would be financially devastating for the home to improve its care by, for example, hiring more staff. This is never an excuse for poor care.

A report by the National Citizens' Coalition for Nursing Home Reform examined the enormous cost to residents and to taxpayers of the inappropriate use of restraints and other substandard care practices. The report found that poor care leads to pressure sores, incontinence and hospitalization. It is very costly to redress the effects of poor nursing home care. Moreover, poor care is physically devastating for residents, who suffer its painful and often permanent effects. Once a resident's condition declines, it is not likely to recover, requiring increasingly heavier care from staff as the resident grows more and more dependent. Chapter 8 reviews these issues in more detail.

Step Up, Speak Up, and Advocate for Good Care

Nursing home residents have a right to quality care that respects their dignity and individual preferences. When problems arise, advocates must step in on behalf of those who can't speak up for themselves. And, they must support those residents who are able to stand up for their rights.

Remember to:

- know the nursing home's complaint process
- determine the specific problem
- decide what you want the outcome to be

- involve friends and/or family members in the process whenever possible
- locate help outside the nursing home.

> — *All laws are subject to change. Regardless of any changes in the federal law discussed in this chapter, these standards are supported in some state laws as well as professional codes of conduct. They are good practice! They represent good care! As a family member you have every right to ask for and expect these practices for your relative.* —

Chapter 8

Why Nursing Homes Are As They Are... and What You Can Do About It

Never doubt that a small group of thoughtful committed citizens can change the world; indeed, it's the only thing that ever does.
— Margaret Mead

EVEN IF YOU DO EVERYTHING THIS BOOK SAYS TO DO, You may still find yourself at a loss. After all, the problems in nursing homes are enormous, complicated and deeply rooted. Throughout this book you've read examples of good care from all over the country. There are thousands of nursing home staff providing good care. Nevertheless, problems continue. In this final chapter, we'll take a look at why these problems persist and how things can change, thanks to *federal and state law, professional development and educational activities* by the nursing home associations, the problem-solving interventions of the *ombudsman program*, and the activism of *concerned consumers*.

Most change comes *one resident at a time*. Indeed, most family advocates don't have the energy to participate in broader efforts. It may be all you can do to support your own family member. In fact, *that's a vital contribution!* Your support for your relative helps the broad-scale advocacy effort. By getting involved for your relative, you're standing up for how things ought to be. Your interventions may improve care for everyone, especially residents who don't have family to stand up for them. Other families may be inspired by your efforts to join you in

> — It may be all you can do to support your own family member. In fact, that's a vital contribution! —

working for changes. Nursing home staff may appreciate your participation and willingness to work together to improve care. Each of these conversations has the potential to change care in your relative's nursing home.

Why Do Nursing Home Problems Persist?

Decade after decade, government agencies, news reporters, and consumer advocates identify problems in nursing home care. At the same time, pioneering health professionals are learning new, more compassionate and effective practices. So, why is there unevenness in the quality of care, even within a single community? Why do problems persist despite one initiative after another to correct them?

At the root of most problems in nursing homes are money, politics, and lack of leadership by management.

Money and Politics. Nursing homes are big business — and getting bigger. In 1999, the United States spent over $68 billion to pay for nursing home care for 1.5 million people. Medicaid pays sixty percent of this amount, which makes Medicaid one of the biggest items in each state's budget. It is a significant factor in the overall national economy, and — at an average private pay cost of $30,000 – $40,000 per year — a significant factor in the economic well-being of individual families.

There is a continual tug of war between the business interests of nursing home proprietors, who want to increase nursing home profits, and the interests of those who pay the bills — governments and families — who want to contain or lower costs.

Time after time, discussions of quality care revert to debates about money. "We would if we could but the state doesn't pay us enough," nursing homes typically say.

Faced with spiraling expenditures and shrinking tax revenues, states constrain the Medicaid budget and then back away from enforcing nursing home regulations.

Where Does the Money Go? Cuts in public funding are not the whole story.

Financial decisions affect resources available for resident care. Nursing home corporations can find profit in many corners. For instance, they may trade properties and speculate about expansions. They may pay high fees to related companies, or subsidiaries that provide management, dietary or other services to the nursing homes they own. Others may use their nursing home properties as financial leverage for real estate or other business ventures. In these same companies, nurse assistants and other staff are usually poorly paid and working with few benefits.

It is not uncommon for a new corporate owner to purchase a facility and make cuts in housekeeping, laundry, or dietary staff, assuring consumers that these cuts won't reduce *nursing* staff. But the nursing staff must pick up the slack in all those departments, contending with soiled linens and dirty floors, transporting trays of food, and assuming other duties — all the while trying to stay on top of their health care responsibilities.

How can a multi-million dollar corporation be out of linen, be short-staffed, or be unable to serve fresh fruits and vegetables? It's a question of leadership, priorities, and public commitment to something better. That's where politics come in.

Politics. There will continue to be wide variation in the quality of nursing home services as long as it is politically and socially acceptable for nursing homes to operate as they do. What is politics if it is not the voice of the public? In the case of nursing homes, making good standards the norm depends on a public expectation of and demand for good care.

Consumer Expectations. Recall the exercise in chapter 1 which asked "What would you need the nursing home to be like to feel okay about living there?" Remember how difficult it was to picture yourself living in a nursing home? Isn't that because you can't help but expect to experience all those losses? When consumers expect nursing home staff to take their individuality into account and offer staff relevant personal information, there is a greater likelihood the home will use that information in caring for residents. That same expectation will carry over into enforcement of public laws about nursing home care.

Consumers Have Strength in Numbers. If you feel as if you're the only family member with concerns, you may hesitate to speak up. As families share experiences, they can join together to support good work going on in the nursing home or raise concerns with a united voice. It's important to understand that millions of other families have faced this dilemma and struggled to find ways to support their relatives. In their efforts, some of them joined others in family groups or outside organizations. Collectively, they have a stronger voice in advocating for good nursing home care.

Ombudsman Programs Need Public Support. Ombudsmen can resolve individual or facility-wide problems and support residents and families who speak out individually or in groups. To be effective, ombudsmen need to have a regular presence in facilities. That takes resources, even when programs rely heavily on trained volunteers. Effectiveness also depends on the willingness of nursing home staff to work cooperatively once concerns are raised. Sometimes ombudsmen must depend on organized family and community concern to convince a nursing home to rethink its practices. Other times ombudsmen must rely on enforcement agencies to ensure that care requirements are met.

Surveyors Are in homes for a Brief Time. Sometimes survey agencies give good ratings to a nursing home, even when the consumer experience at the home is poor. Generally the home is prepared for the arrival of the surveyors. Surveyors may lack the time to develop sufficient documentation to support a finding of poor care. Nursing homes may opt to take a survey agency to court before correcting cited problems. Consumers often complain that surveyors don't cite real problems because a situation wasn't documented in the record or wasn't directly observed by the surveyor. Some survey agencies have not made the shift in thinking — away from paper compliance — to support and promote good individualized care practices.

It's a Matter of Leadership
When nursing home owners and administrators have a commitment to quality, they lead in a way that supports good care. Today, many American businesses and government agencies are using ideas of "quality" to improve management practices. *Total Quality Management or Continuous Quality Improvement* principles maintain that:
 • The most cost effective way to do something is to *do it right the first time,* with as little waste as possible.

• To do something right, businesses must be in *continual contact with their customers* to determine what consumers need and how well business is meeting their needs.

• Businesses also must have *open communication with their front-line staff,* who can tell them what is needed to get the job done well.

How does this relate to nursing homes? Look at each of these management principles again.

Do It Right the First Time. There's a high cost to poor care! While nursing home care is costly to provide, it is more cost effective to give good care.

The references to chemical and physical restraint use in this book give ample examples to support this contention. If residents are able to walk, why over-medicate them so they can't walk? If facilities restrain residents rather than support their activity, what are the consequences? How soon will they lose their ability to walk, to stand, to go the toilet? How long before they cannot bathe, eat, or dress themselves? How much does it cost to care for their induced incontinence or for skin sores caused by sitting for long periods of time in soiled clothes? We already know that encouraging independence is basic to good care. With good assessment and care planning, staff can identify the underlying causes of problems and approach care constructively and effectively.

Maintain Continual Contact with Consumers. In nursing homes, this means having an individualized approach to care. Without continual consultation with the consumer, or the resident, staff's efforts often are counterproductive. Too often staff react to the *symptoms* instead of getting to the *cause* of the problem.

When nursing home staff rush to quiet a resident's agitation, instead of listening to it and looking for its source, they aren't listening to the customer. When staff contain a resident's distress instead of investigating it, they make more work for themselves in the long run. The solutions to residents' needs are often readily available. Conducting individualized assessment and care planning, knowing the person, observing responses — these are the staff efforts that provide clues for care strategies.

This book began by talking about the fear so many people have about losing their individuality and their identity when they enter a nursing home. An essential element of good management is *knowing* each individual consumer. By using that knowledge, nursing homes can provide good care, tailored to individual needs and preferences.

Maintain Open Communication with Staff. The third ingredient to good management is effective involvement and input from staff. Nursing home administrators who excuse problems by lamenting the difficulty of getting good staff are simply conceding poor leadership and management. Nurse assistants, who provide ninety percent of the hands-on care in nursing homes, are generally left out of all critical decision-making. They seldom attend a care-planning meeting, or contribute to a care-planning discussion. Many never see a resident's care plan or discuss how to achieve the care goals for that resident.

Instead, nurse assistants clean up the soiled clothes when residents are restrained in geri-chairs. They deal with residents' restlessness, agitation and boredom when residents aren't engaged in meaningful activities. And, nurse assistants receive the brunt of residents' depression and distress when social workers are not able to attend to residents' psychosocial needs.

In contrast, nursing home leaders who create a good place to live for residents are also creating a good place to work. A home that permanently assigns staff to work regularly with the same residents is supporting the relationships needed for individualized care, and reducing turnover and absenteeism at the same time. These nursing staff have the support of professional nurses.

While it's important to have enough money to provide good service, even more crucial is how that money is used. Corporate owners who opt to invest their money in real estate and other financial ventures, rather than investing in staff development and resources, compromise resident care. Strong, collaborative leadership can motivate staff to find innovative solutions to even the most complicated and daunting care dilemmas. But first, everyone — from the top down — must agree that solutions are attainable and worth pursuing.

Money, Management and Leadership — The Way It Can Be

Joyce Steier described to the U.S. Senate Special Committee on Aging, October 22, 1990, how she introduced a program of restorative care in her nursing home and changed the caregiving and workplace culture:

I'm the administrator of a 180-bed facility in Largo, Florida. We are a for-profit organization and my boss makes it very clear... that I must keep that in mind... I am a new administrator to this facility... This facility had a census of 110 — so we had seventy empty beds that were generating no revenue...

We began the program very slowly and certainly got the rehab nursing program going. That was finding out if there were limbs that could be moved that hadn't been moved in a long time. Our physical therapy department and our occupational therapy offered a lot of assistance to us and to the staff. They did a lot of training. But the majority of the work was done by the nursing department and by the regular staff...

... You have to learn to use the staff that you have there in your building. I have housekeepers that walk down corridors every day on their way to lunch, and now they take a resident or two along with them. We have utilized the maintenance department, the activities, the social service, and everyone else in the facility to help us get this program going. They are not used as often as they were before because a lot of our residents have learned to walk, so it's not necessary to use them.

But in the beginning I urge you to get all the people in your facility involved in this. I think that the more people you have the less overwhelming it seems.

In the last three months things have really changed since we have put this program in. First of all — the thing that makes any corporation very happy — is that we now have 160 residents...

I think the morale of the staff has dramatically changed. They feel a part of the program. I think that from the housekeepers and the laundry people to the nurse assistants and the nurses — they feel like we're all committed to achieve a common goal. I think that's the part that makes things seem better to them. That's why we have less turnover.

We have certainly eliminated buying restraints, wheelchairs, geri-chairs, and all those things that you always buy in nursing homes that are very expensive. Another benefit is that the residents are eating so much better. I think moving them around and giving them a chance to sit at a dining room table in a chair rather than in their wheelchair or having difficulty reaching their food has made a significant difference...

One of the other benefits for the company, and certainly for the residents, has been that we buy less incontinence supplies. We have decreased the amount of diapers and under-pads, which are also very costly, by about thirty percent.

We have certainly decreased and reduced the potential for developing decubitus ulcers. I think if any of you are nurses in the audience, you know how time consuming and how costly treating them is in any facility.

As a result of this program, one of the other good things that happened is that we had to take a long look at chemical restraints because you can't untie people and ambulate them around if you're going to sedate them at medicine time. So we've had to decrease that tremendously...

I believe that you can change the duties of what any of your employees do, reduce your agency bill, increase morale, and still operate within the restrictions of a budget. As you increase profit and the census goes up, a wonderful thing happens. When you start giving good care, it seems like the whole world hears about it, and particularly that world that surrounds your nursing home... We now have a waiting list... They've heard about the good things that are happening at Oak Manor.

Quality Care is Good for Staff, Too

This program of restorative care improved care for residents and had a positive affect on the staff. Staff felt better about coming to work everyday. Staff need caring work environments to help them do their job.

Staffing Shortages. Nursing homes have trouble attracting and keeping staff because of the low pay, poor benefits, difficult working conditions, and poor management. Efforts are underway in many states and nationally to invest more resources in staffing and draw more good people into caregiving work.

Quality Jobs. While pay and benefits are important, the quality of the work environment also makes a big difference. A project in Massachusetts[1] helps nursing homes transition from a *culture of* turnover to a culture of *staff* retention by improving caregiving and workplace practices.[2]

The caregiving connection between residents and certified nurse assistants is the foundation for quality care. Maintaining and supporting this connection requires changes in nursing home practice.

---

[1] Funded through the FY 01 Nursing Home Quality Initiative spearheaded by Senator Mark Montigny.

[2] For more information on direct care worker issues, contact the Paraprofessional Healthcare Institute at www.paraprofessional.org and www.directcareclearinghouse.org.

Nursing Homes need to transition from a culture of high staff turnover and poor care to a culture of staff retention and good care by:

1. Establishing consistent assignment so that aides work every day with the same residents. They can get to know each other and establish relationships that can be the basis for kind caregiving.
2. Using supportive and inclusive supervisory and management practices that foster team work and shared problem solving.
3. Bringing continuing education into the workplace to improve workers' skills and provide opportunities for career development.
4. Paying living wages, providing health insurance and other important benefits that give workers economic security.
5. Maintaining staffing ratios that allow staff enough time to meet residents' quality of care and quality of life needs. See NCCNHR web site for information on staffing, www.nursinghomeaction.org.

A number of nursing homes around the country have pioneered new caregiving and workplace practices that improve the quality of care for residents and the quality of the job for staff.

Making It Happen

The Nursing Home Reform law makes quality the standard of care and gives consumers recourse if nursing homes provide poor care. The law came after twenty years of public discussion about the need for better nursing home care. It drew on professional standards of practice for nursing, medicine, social work, and other fields. It came about because of intensive advocacy by concerned consumers, progressive providers, and committed public policy makers. Use the knowledge that individualized care promotes well-being in daily advocacy for your relative. Public demand for good assessment, care planning and care delivery is one of the most important steps toward ensuring that nursing homes provide care and services that respect residents' individual needs and help them maintain their function.

About the Law

Laws, of course, reflect the political and social times, and are subject to change. Changes in the standards of the Nursing Home Reform Law have been and continue to be, proposed in Congress. Changes driven by fiscal constraints are virtually certain to affect the quality of care and life for nursing home residents. It's imperative that consumers like you monitor the proposed changes in both federal and state laws on nursing home care. Because you have a relative in a nursing home, you are the most potent force in continuing to improve care in nursing homes. Your relative, as well as other residents, are dependent upon you to keep speaking up for quality of care and quality of life on their behalf. Your State Long Term Care Ombudsman or the National Citizens' Coalition for Nursing Home Reform can give you information about the status of federal and state laws. Contact information for each of these is in Appendix 7.

Remember, too, that the standards established by the 1987 law are widely accepted as guidelines for good practice in nursing homes.

What Can You Do? Summing It Up

Throughout this book, we've described the role you can play in the effort to put good standards of care into practice on behalf of your relative/resident. Here's a brief summary of what you can do:

• **Respect the dignity and rights of your relative.** Support your relative's efforts to control her life and help give voice to her choices and desires. Remember that a person with dementia may not always express responses or preferences in conventional ways, but may still let you know if she's uneasy or uncomfortable. You may be able to recognize signs that others can't. Unusual agitation or aggression is probably a sign of distress. Help staff interpret actions and respond to the unmet need rather than suppress the symptoms.

• **Provide information about your relative.** What have been your relative's interests during his life? What has calmed his agitation in recent years? What are his habits and patterns in the morning, in the evening, and throughout the day? What gives him satisfaction or pleasure? (See Appendix 4.) How does he seem to be responding to life at the home?

• **Ask questions and be involved. Work with nursing home staff to support good care for the person you love.** If staff have chosen a particular course of action, ask for more information. What are the consequences? What are the alternatives?

• **Seek support from staff, such as the director of nursing, the social worker, or the resident assessment coordinator.** These staff can be a link for you in trying to resolve concerns within the home. Explain your relative's needs, interpret his responses if staff need to understand him better. Ask their help in communicating with others responsible for providing care.

• **Learn about the contents of the current federal and state laws and regulations and professional standards for good nursing home care.** Use these as a guide in asking questions about care. Participate in family meetings with staff when care issues come up. Ask for more information if you notice a decline. Discuss care options and their consequences. Help the law work for your relative.

• **Learn about the Long-Term Care Ombudsman Program and citizens groups that can assist consumers in resolving nursing home problems.** Perhaps you can volunteer, even in a small way, to support their efforts. You may have the time, now or in the future, to be a volunteer for the Ombudsman Program and/or join a citizen advocacy group. You can advocate for residents who have no family to look after their interests.

• **Tell the surveyors what you've experienced when they make their annual inspection of the home.** Give a full range of your experiences with as much detail as possible so surveyors can use your information in their evaluation of the home. They can protect your confidentiality if you ask them.

• **Share your experiences and support others who are working for change.** If you can't make a substantial commitment, you may be able to help by providing information or assistance as the ombudsman assigned to your home looks into and attempts to resolve problems other residents face. You might give testimony before the state legislature when lawmakers consider changes in nursing home laws or reimbursement. Or, you may opt to assist others who share your concerns and are working to make the system work for their relative in the nursing home.

In the end, it's your efforts on behalf of your relative that will make the most difference. Our intimate ties of family and friendship are the mainstay of our lives. Your honest efforts to maintain this important connection, and your openness in hearing the conflicts and heartaches of nursing home life, can give the person you love a real, caring relationship, when so much else about the integrity of her life is at risk. You may not always be able to change care practices or make the system work. But sometimes you will. Your individual effort is the first line of defense for the person you love. This can be truly overwhelming. Don't carry the burden alone. Reach out to other family members and friends. Reach out to state, local and national organizations for support. Talk to them about what you see and what you've learned.

Remember that people feel worse when they feel powerless and isolated. That's how so many nursing home residents feel. Let them know they are *not* alone. You are there. And know, too, that you are not without help. Reach out for it through the information and resources identified in this book. Even if you aren't able to make major changes at your nursing home, your advocacy will surely give comfort to your relative. It will offer hope to others who share your experiences!

• **Join the National Citizens' Coalition for Nursing Home Reform.** To obtain information, contact them at the address given in Appendix 7, page 149.

Appendix 1
Glossary

Contracture

Temporary or permanent shortening of muscles; left untreated, can cause a resident's body to curl up, with arms pressed tight to sides, like an infant in a fetal position.

Feeding tube

Tube inserted through nose to stomach, or directly into the stomach or intestine, for purpose of administering nutrition.

Geri-chair

A wheelchair that cannot be self-propelled and must be pushed by someone else. It has a high back, foot ledge and a removable dining tray. It is a restraint.

Immobility

Inability to move around without help.

Incontinence

Inability to control bladder or bowel movements; resident wets or soils.

Pressure Sore

Persistent red spot on the skin; can also be a break in the skin, deep sore, or crater-like wound; found, most commonly, on the end of spine (coccyx); also found on the hips, heels, elbows, shoulders, and, in rare cases, the ears.

Range-of-Motion Exercises

Daily exercise to maintain joint and muscle flexibility. Resident may do them alone or with the aid of staff.

Transferring

Movement back and forth from bed to chair, wheelchair, toilet, etc.

Urinary catheter

Flexible tube inserted into body cavity or vessel to remove urine when bladder no longer functions.

Appendix 2
Standard of Nursing Home Care

The standard of care is set by federal and state laws and regulations and by what is known to be good practice within health care professions.

The standard of care is embodied in the phrase that facilities provide "care and services to attain the highest possible physical, mental and psychosocial well-being of each resident."

It has four features: Do no harm; maximize resident's well-being; respect their informed consent; attend to quality of life as well as the quality of care.

- As is true in all medical care, the first principle guiding the standard of care is *to do no harm. This means that no harm should come to someone because of the actions taken by the nursing home staff.*

> *For example, if a person was able to walk when she entered the facility, the nursing home staff should not do anything that will make her unable to walk.*

The same is true of other resident abilities. A resident "should not decline" in his ability to dress, eat, bathe, or remain continent, and his state of mind should not deteriorate.

Of course, sometimes it is impossible to prevent deterioration. Sometimes the decline is caused by:
- the onset of a new condition.
  For example, your father may have been walking just fine but then suffer a stroke and no longer be able to walk.
- the natural progression of an existing condition.
  For example, your mother's Alzheimer's disease might progress so that she is unable to care for herself in ways she was able to when she was first admitted.
- a resident's refusal of treatment.
  For example, your grandmother may just give up on eating at a certain point and be ready to face her end, or your diabetic uncle may choose not to have a limb amputated even though it will mean a more rapid deterioration from diabetes.

When this deterioration occurs, the professional standard of care calls for nursing home staff to do what they can to:
- slow the decline by looking for risk factors and working to prevent their occurrence.
  For example, after your father's stroke limits his mobility, he may be at risk for skin breakdown or muscle contractures. The staff should help him shift position and keep moving his limbs.
- assisting the resident to maintain as much function and independence as possible within the declining condition.

For example, your mother's dementia may make her more disoriented. The staff should find ways for her to continue to walk around, but help her to do so safely.

• The second guiding principle is to *maximize people's well-being by helping people recover* from an illness or condition, as much as is possible. This means you can expect nursing home staff to identify areas where recovery is possible and provide any necessary therapy or assistance.

For example, after your father's stroke, the nursing home should provide whatever therapy (physical, occupational, speech, etc.) will help him regain function and should provide substitutes to enable him to continue to function, such as language boards to assist with communication.

Nursing home staff conduct an assessment of the resident's abilities, limitations and areas of risk to determine how to help each resident "attain or maintain" his highest possible well-being. Through this assessment, staff identify potential areas for improvement in function and areas in which the resident is at risk for decline or is actually declining.

• As staff design a plan of care to help residents maintain strengths and slow the progress of their decline, residents are entitled to attend these care conferences and to have family with them so that they can make informed decisions about their care. This is called *informed consent* and is another principle standard of care. Informed consent means that no treatment should be administered without a person's full agreement. In order to give full agreement, you would need to know all the options and their risks and benefits. In nursing homes that means that the staff need to let residents and their families know what health care problems they wish to address, what options they have for addressing them and the pro's and con's of each option. Remember: *People don't lose the right to make decisions about their health care treatment when they move into a nursing home.*

• Resident and family participation is important because there are so many personal factors that affect how someone responds to care. These are often referred to as *"quality of life issues."* This standard of care means that it is as important to attend to the spirit as it is to attend to the body. Nursing homes need to help people feel respected, support their dignity, accommodate their individual needs and encourage and assist their participation in decisions of significance to them.

Appendix 3
Resident's Rights

A Summary of the Major Provisions of the 1987 Nursing Home Reform Law

I. The Right to Be Fully Informed
1. The right to be informed of all services available and all charges.
2. The right to a copy of the facility's rules and regulations.
3. The right to be informed of the address and telephone number of the State Ombudsman, the State licensure office and other advocacy groups and the facility shall post these numbers.
4. The right to see the State survey reports on the facility.
5. The right to daily communication in their language and the right to assistance if there is sensory impairment.

II. The Right to Participate In Their Own Care
1. The right to receive adequate or appropriate health care.
2. The right to be informed of their medical condition and to participate in treatment planning: The resident and their representative shall be invited to participate in care planning.
3. The right to refuse medication and treatment.
4. The right to participate in discharge planning.
5. The right to review their medical records.

III. The Right to Make Independent Choices
1. The right to know that choices are available.
2. The right to make independent personal decisions.
3. The right to choose their own physician.
4. The right to participate in activities of the community inside and outside the facility.
5. The right to vote.
6. The right to participate in a Resident Council.

IV. The Right to Privacy and Confidentiality
1. The right to private and unrestricted communication with any person of their choice, including: privacy for telephone calls; unopened mail; privacy for meetings with family and friends and other residents.
2. The right to privacy in treatment and caring for their personal needs.
3. The facility must provide reasonable access to any entity or individual that provides health, social, legal or other services.
4. The right to confidentiality regarding their medical, personal or financial affairs.

V. The Right to Dignity, Respect and Freedom
1. The right to be treated with consideration, respect and with the fullest measure of dignity.
2. The right to be free from mental and physical abuse.
3. The right to be free from physical and chemical restraints.
4. The right to self-determination.

VI. The Right to Security for Their Possessions
1. The right to manage their own financial affairs.
2. The right to file a complaint with the State survey and certification agency for abuse, neglect or misappropriation of their property.

VII. The Right to Remain in the Facility
1. The right to be transferred or discharged only for medical reasons, for their welfare if their needs cannot be met in the facility, if the health and safety of other residents is endangered, or for non-payment of stay.
2. The right to receive notice of transfer. A thirty-day notice for transfer out of the facility must be given. The notice must include the reason for transfer, the effective date, the location to which the resident is discharged, a statement of right to appeal, the name, address and telephone number of the state long- term care ombudsman.
3. The facility must provide sufficient preparation of residents to ensure a safe transfer or discharge.

VIII. The Right to Raise Concerns or Complaints
1. The right to present grievances for themselves or others to the staff of the nursing home, or to any other person, without fear of reprisal.
2. The right to prompt efforts by the facility to resolve grievances.

IX. The facility must maintain identical policies and practices regarding transfer, discharge and the provision of services for all individuals regardless of payment source.

Appendix 4
"I Want To Tell You About My Mother...."

A Guide to Providing Helpful Information to Nursing Home Staff
Developed by Carter Catlett Williams, MSW, ACSW, Consultant

When a person enters a nursing home an important and valuable part of the experience is to talk to staff about herself and what life has been like. However, many individuals may have to rely on their families to give such information for them.

All of us have the stories of our relatives' lives inside us. These stories are so much a part of us and our own lives that we hardly know where to begin. We aren't used to stepping back a little to see our parents' lives in their wholeness. We're more used to exchanging much-loved anecdotes about mother, father, aunt, or uncle, in family gatherings.

To introduce your relative to nursing home staff, helping them know who this person is, is one of the most important things you can do! It will rescue your relative from the limbo of being in strange surroundings where *"nobody knows who I am."* It'll make all the difference in staff understanding your relative's actions and responses because they will know some of the thoughts, feelings, habits and life experiences that lie behind those actions and responses.

But where to start and what to include? There are the easy-to- recite concrete facts that the social worker, or other staff, will request at admission time. Then there is your relative's unique life story that you'll want to be sure the staff knows as well. Both are necessary for staff to come to know your relative. In addition, this is the appropriate time to describe to staff what kind of day makes a good day for this particular person.

To illustrate the type of information you'll want to give staff, look at the following outline. It might give you ideas about other details to include. *Assume your mother is being admitted.*

- **Facts:** Tell about your mother's:
  Birth date and place
  Number of sisters and brothers; where your mother falls in the birth order; number of sisters and brothers still living
  Rural or urban childhood
  Your mother's ethnic community
  Schooling
  Marriage and date of marriage
  Children
  Employment outside of home before and after marriage
  Religious affiliation
  Hobbies

Date of divorce or widowhood
Living arrangements during marriage and afterwards
Reason for entering the nursing home.

- **Story:** A person's story includes hopes, aspirations, and accomplishments, as well as disappointments, losses, and the things that didn't go so well. It includes the person's characteristic ways of handling the ups and downs of life. Here are some suggestions to help you think over your mother's life and tell her story.
  What she looked forward to in life: as a child, as a teenager
  How much she was able to realize her dreams
  If she had a career outside home and family, what the career meant to her
  How she and her family coped with the Great Depression of the 1930's
  How World Wars I and II affected her life, as well as the Korean and
      Vietnam wars
  What she wanted for her children
  Her relationships with her family
  Whether religious faith was important to her and how she expresses that:
      prayer, reading scripture, attendance at church, synagogue, or mosque,
      volunteer activity, helping others in the community
  What she had, and now has, the most fun doing: cooking for the family;
      hosting family gatherings; gardening; singing; reading; fishing; playing
      bingo; handwork; going to the movies; sports as a player or spectator;
      enjoying nature; seeing family and old friends
  Whether she likes to crack jokes or enjoys other's jokes
  How she handled money
  Whether she had pets and what they meant to her
  What angers her
  What pleases her
  What saddens her
  What comforts her
  Whether she generally has an optimistic attitude or tends to see more the
      dark side of things
  Her major satisfactions and disappointments
  What she values most in life
  What you value most about her
To add further richness to your mother's story, collect photographs in an album for her room and take others to hang on her walls.

- What Makes a Good Day for your mother, covering:
  Daily schedule
      When she likes to get up and go to bed, times of rest and quiet
      How she prefers to spend her day
      What her mornings and evenings are like at home

Times of her favorite radio and/or TV programs
When and what she likes for snacks
When and how often she likes to go outside
Her usual bowel and bladder patterns
Her patterns with: bathing, eating, and food preferences
The particular things that give her satisfaction and pleasure
Particular foods at certain meals
Careful grooming in the style she prefers
The chance to be alone at least some part of each day
Activities she enjoys: music, movies
Attendance at worship service or other expression of her faith
Where she prefers to place things in her room and at her bedside
How she typically expresses affection and is comfortable receiving
affection: hugs? kisses? touching?

Remember no detail is too small if it's significant to your relative!

• **For Men:** If your relative is a man, the same type of information as previously listed is equally important. In addition, you need to be sure that activities and the response of staff consider things from a man's perspective. More physical outlets or more traditionally masculine pursuits might need to be offered for your relative.

Appendix 5
Check List for Evaluating a Nursing Home

Here is a check list of items which may help you evaluate a nursing home, whether you're choosing one or learning how to make things work in the home where a family member resides.

Any nursing home you visit will probably not meet *all* these expectations. The presence or absence of any of the items does not automatically mean that the facility is excellent or poor. Some have strong points in one area, others in another. What you must consider are the needs of the resident or potential resident, then decide what is most important to that person and to you. It may be that the most important thing to both of you is that the home be close to your residence so that you can visit often without a long drive.

In visiting a nursing home, you don't have to be an inspector! Most family members, as well as ombudsmen, say they can tell a great deal about a home just from watching the interaction of staff and residents. Is the conversation happy, cheerful and respectful? The check list includes the question, *"What makes a day good for you?"* Although this open-ended question doesn't have a *correct* answer, the way residents answer this will give you some ideas about the home. For instance, if a resident tells you no day is good or you hear that every day is good, you'll have some clues about how residents feel about living there. Other responses may provide some helpful information about daily life.

If nursing homes feel like a foreign country to you, take a friend along who can help. If at all possible, take the potential resident with you, at least for one visit! Just seeing a nursing home from the inside can help alleviate a person's fear.

This list is just one more piece of information to add to your observations, conversations with others who know the facility, and other information you gather. For comparisons between nursing homes, it may be helpful to check the strong and weak points for each item and each home. Visit each home more than once and at different times if at all possible.

Many people don't have enough time to shop for a nursing home because medical circumstances require quick action. Or your relative may already be in a nursing home. These items can assist you in raising issues with nursing home staff and learning more about how the nursing home works so you have a better idea of what you can do to have the situation work best for your relative.

The questions on the check list are more thoroughly discussed throughout this book. In order to more accurately assess a facility on each of these, *IT IS IMPORTANT TO READ THIS BOOK.*

Check List for Evaluating a Nursing Home

A. Using your senses: sight, hearing, smell, touch   **Strong**   **Weak**

1. Is there cheerful, respectful, pleasant, warm interaction
   between staff and residents?   _____   _____
2. Does the administrator seem to know the residents and
   enjoy being with them?   _____   _____
3. Do staff and administration seem comfortable with
   each other?   _____   _____
4. Do the rooms appear to reflect the individuality of their
   occupants? Do all of the rooms look alike?   _____   _____
5. Are residents using the common rooms — for example,
   the front lounge?   _____   _____
6. What is the noise level in the facility? Is it comfortable
   and homelike? Are there quiet places for residents?   _____   _____
7. Do residents look clean and well groomed?   _____   _____
8. Is the home free from unpleasant odors?   _____   _____
9. Do you notice a swift response to call lights?   _____   _____
10. Are there residents crying out? If so,do they get an
    appropriate response from staff?   _____   _____
11. Is the dining room atmosphere relaxed and conducive
    to pleasant meals?   _____   _____
12. Do the meals look appetizing? Are residents eating most
    of their food? Do they have assistance if they need it?   _____   _____
13. Does the home seem clean, cheerful, uncrowded?   _____   _____
14. Are there pleasant areas for family visits?   _____   _____
15. Are there residents in physical restraints? (See chapter 5.) _____   _____
16. Do residents appear to be engaged in meaningful activity
    by themselves or with others? (as opposed to staring at
    the wall, blaring TV, slumped over, or in a line)   _____   _____

B. Things you can ask of staff

1. What kinds of activities are residents involved in?
   Is there access to books, gardening, community activities,
   pets, to retain linkages to former interests? Does the
   nursing home have a wheelchair accessible van?   _____   _____
2. What kind of activities are there for residents with
   dementia? (structured, walking paths, evening activities,
   music?)   _____   _____
3. Is there permanent assignment of staff to residents?   _____   _____
4. How are the nurse assistants involved in the resident's
   care planning process? (They should attend and
   contribute ideas.)   _____   _____

	Strong	Weak

5. How does the staff accommodate the family's schedule to assure participation in care planning meetings? _____ _____

6. What happens if a resident refuses to take a medication? _____ _____

7. What does the facility do for residents who are depressed? Is counseling available? _____ _____

8. What is the facility policy toward missing clothing and other possessions? _____ _____

9. What does the facility do to encourage employee retention and continuity? Does the staff receive health benefits? _____ _____

10. Does the facility provide transportation to community activities? _____ _____

11. What kinds of therapies are provided for residents on Medicaid? (Occupational therapy, speech therapy, physical therapy, mental health services, etc.) _____ _____

12. Is there a family council? Are there family members I can speak to? _____ _____

13. What happens when someone has a problem or complaint? Are family/staff conferences available to work out problems? _____ _____

14. Who is your ombudsman? Does that person visit regularly? _____ _____

15. What are the extra charges not included in the daily rate? _____ _____

16. (If you pay privately) How often have private pay rates increased? How much notice is given before an increase? Are there charges for extra care which are not included in the daily rate? _____ _____

17. What do staff see as the facility's main strengths and weakness? _____ _____

18. Who decides for each resident how she bathes and how often? _____ _____

19. Who selects roommates? What do you consider in selecting roommates? How are residents involved in the selection? _____ _____

20. How are smokers and non-smokers accommodated? _____ _____

C. Things you can learn from residents and families

1. What is your usual routine? Can you get up and go to bed when you wish? _____ _____

2. Do you have the same nurse assistant most days? (Does this match the answer to B3?) _____ _____

3. Are snacks available when you want one? Are they what you want? _____ _____

	Strong	Weak
4. Do you participate in care planning meetings? Is your opinion valued? (Does this match the answer to B5?)	_____	_____
5. Are care planning conferences held at a time when family members can attend? Do the conferences last until your questions are answered or all of the issues have been taken care of?	_____	_____
6. What happens when you have missing clothing? (Does this match the answer to B8?)	_____	_____
7. Are residents able to get help for going to the toilet within a short period of time?	_____	_____
8. Whom do you go to with problems? What is the response? Are you satisfied?	_____	_____
9. How do staff help you with your personal interests like reading or gardening?	_____	_____
10. Do you get outside as often as you wish?	_____	_____
11. Is there a resident council? How does it work? Who controls the council: residents or staff?	_____	_____
12. Is there a family council? Is it an effective forum for raising concerns and learning what's happening at the home?	_____	_____
13. What's the best thing about living here?	_____	_____
14. What's the worst thing about living here?	_____	_____
15. What makes a day good for you?	_____	_____

D. Information you can obtain

	Strong	Weak
1. Copy of state inspection report-either from the agency which licenses and certifies nursing homes, from the facility itself, or from the ombudsman.	_____	_____
2. Information about the facility from the local ombudsman or state ombudsman.	_____	_____
3. Information from family members or friends of residents.	_____	_____

Appendix 6
[A] Good Care Prevents Poor Outcomes

Preventable Poor Outcomes

Preventive Care

Bladder or bowel incontinence due to immobility or poor memory.

Nursing home staff must take resident to toilet, according to individualized care plan and upon resident's request.

Use of urinary catheter due to inadequate toileting.

Toilet as noted above. Use of restorative care. Use adult incontinent brief only as adjunct to toileting. Residents shouldn't be told to relieve themselves in their clothing because incontinent brief is on. Catheters can be used appropriately only when: obtaining sterile urine specimen; removing urine from bladder in the event of nerve damage; and trying to heal a skin wound.

Malnutrition/dehydration due to immobility, inability to understand or remember.

Provide nourishing food that resident enjoys. Assist with eating, per care plan. Family and friends can help, especially if resident takes a long time to eat.

Tube feedings because staff is too busy to help residents feed themselves.

Same as above. Never accept "she takes too long to eat" as adequate reason for tube feedings. Inserting a tube through the nose into the stomach, or directly into the stomach, is an uncomfortable invasive procedure that seriously diminishes quality of life. You should ask, "Would I want to endure that?"

Preventable Poor Outcomes

Resident poorly dressed and groomed. Mouth and foot care poor due to busy staff, poorly trained staff, or poor staff supervision.

Pressure sores due to: immobility; poor nutrition; poor fluid intake; incontinence.

Contractures due to immobility.

Decreased independence; loss of ability to dress, groom, eat, toilet, etc. Caused by lack of restorative services, treatments.

Preventive Care

Staff should help resident to groom and dress as needed. Clothes should be clean, though spills can occur during meals and activities. Staff should help keep mouth clean, free from food. Feet should be kept clean and dry; use lotion to soften skin; toenails should be filed.

See that staff position the resident at least every two hours; two people should move heavy, immobile resident to avoid friction of sheet against body. Prevention equipment includes: sheepskin booties on heels and elbows; special mattresses; special cushions in wheelchairs. Encourage resident to eat and drink; toilet as needed, keeping skin clean and dry; place pillows between knees, ankles, arms and body; help residents out of bed daily.

Staff should perform range-of-motion exercises for each joint from neck to toes at least daily. Help residents out of bed daily. Position resident in bed or chair with pillows/foam rolls between knees, ankles, arms and body. Residents should not be tilted to one side in a chair.

Staff should provide assistance to promote independence. If resident can eat alone, but takes a long time, staff should not try to feed the resident to save time.

Preventable Poor Outcomes

Preventive Care

Drug interaction due to: too many drugs, wrong types of drugs, and too high dosage.

Staff should reassess drugs to see why they are administered and how they affect residents. Look for: drop in blood pressure that causes residents to fall when they try to stand; dry mouth or skin; poor appetite; upset stomach; vision change; excess urination; restlessness; personality change.

Inability to see or hear due to: lost/broken hearing aids or lost/ dirty/ broken eyeglasses.

Staff should ensure hearing aids/ eyeglasses are operating and kept in safe place.

[B] How Do You Know When Preventive Care is Needed?

At-Risk Residents Are:

Preventable Poor Outcome

Immobile (unable to move without help) due to: injury, disease, drugs or restraints.

Pressure on coccyx (small triangular bone near end of spine), hips, heels, shoulders. Contractures forcing resident into fetal position, curled up with rounded back and bent knees. Bladder and bowel incontinence and possible use of catheter. Malnutrition or poor diet. Dehydration or insufficient fluids.

Non-communicative or unable to be understood due to injury or disease.

Bladder or bowel incontinence and possible use of catheter. Also can result in malnutrition, dehydration and decreased ability to eat, dress, walk and perform other activities of daily living.

Demented or unable to remember due to injury, disease drugs.

Same as above. Also, decreased mobility unrelated to disease, plus increased risk of accidents.

[C] Rehabilitative/Restorative Care to Increase Function

Care Problem	Rehabilitative/ Restorative Care	Who Requires Care?
Incontinence	Bowel and bladder training. Staff should visit with resident every two hours to check whether resident is clean/dry, or needs to go to the toilet. Staff also monitor frequency/amount bladder and bowels excrete. Food and fluid intake also measured.	Residents who can regain control of bladder and bowels, but do not have a bladder infection, severe memory loss, nerve damage to bladder, or bowel disease.
Immobility	Physical therapy (PT) department schedules regular sessions until no further improvement possible. Resident then transfers to preventive maintenance program. Resident learns to stand; pivot; transfer from bed to chair; walk; and use canes, crutches, walkers and wheelchairs.	Residents who lost movement due to falls, broken hip, stroke, improper restraint use, or accidents.
	Restorative range of motion exercises: Over time range of motion may increase.	Resident who has start of contracture due to poor care in past.

Care Problem	Rehabilitative/ Restorative Care	Who Requires Care?
Unable to dress and groom oneself.	Occupational therapist suggest changes in clothes, grooming equipment such as Velcro closures if resident can't button clothes. Breaks down each task so it can be relearned step by step — teaches nurse how to follow with program.	Resident whose loss of function is due to injury or poor care.
Unable to eat/drink independently.	Occupational therapy: Same as above but emphasis on special equipment such as plates with high rim, tableware with built up handles. Dietary: providing appropriate foods; a thickener in liquids if unable to swallow; finger foods for those unable to remember how to use a fork and knife. Speech therapist: assesses swallowing ability and suggests changes in foods, positioning for eating and drinking.	Resident who has lost function due to injury, disease, poor care.

Care Problem	Rehabilitative/ Restorative Care	Who Requires Care?
Ability to communicate	Speech therapist evaluates problem and does exercises to improve speech. When speech *cannot* be regained suggests other communication devices: pencil, paper, electronic devices. Teaches staff to follow through when therapist not there. Audiology services — evaluate residents hearing and prescribes appropriate devices. Staff must keep device in good working order and be sure it is not lost. Optometrist — prescribes glasses. Staff must help to keep devices in good working order and be sure they are not lost.	Residents who have lost hearing or speaking ability due to injury, disease or lost equipment.

Appendix 7
Resources

National Citizens' Coalition for Nursing Home Reform (NCCNHR)
1424 16th St., N.W., #202, Washington, DC 20036
Phone: (202) 332-2275   Fax: (202) 332-2949
E-mail: nccnhr@nccnhr.org   Web site: www.nursinghomeaction.org

Contact NCCNHR for information and other resources:
- A current list of citizen advocacy group(s) in your area;
- NCCNHR publications;
- Membership information;
- Links to other organizations working on long-term care issues.

State Long-Term Care Ombudsman Programs

Alabama Dept. of Senior Services
770 Washington Avenue
RSA Plaza, Suite 470
Montgomery, AL 36130
Phone: (334) 242-5743

Alaska Mental Health Trust Authority
550 West 7th Avenue, Ste. 1830
Anchorage, AK 99501
Phone: (907) 334-4480

Arizona Aging & Adult Administration
1789 West Jefferson 2SW 950A
Phoenix, AZ 85007
Phone: (602) 542-6440

Arkansas Div. of Aging & Adult Serv.
P.O.B. 1437 Slot 1412
Little Rock, AR 72201-1437
Phone: (501) 682-2441

California Department on Aging
1600 K Street
Sacramento, CA 95814
Phone: (916) 324-3968

State Licensure and Certification Programs

Alabama Dept. of Public Health
Div. of Licensure and Certification
PO Box 303017
Montgomery, AL 36130-3017
Phone: (334) 206-5077

Health Facilities Licensing & Certification
4730 Bus. Park Blvd., Suite 18
Anchorage, AK 99503-7137
Phone: (907) 561-8081

Arizona Dept. of Health
Assurance and Licensure
1647 East Morten Ave., #220
Phoenix, AZ 85020
Phone: (602) 674-4200

Arkansas Dept. of Health
Freeway Medical Tower
5800 West 10th St., Suite 400
Little Rock, AR 72204
Phone: (501) 661-2201

California Dept of Health Services
Licensing & Certification Dvsn
1800 3rd Street, #210
Sacramento, CA 94234-7320
Phone: (916) 445-3054

State Ombudsman Programs

Colorado Ombudsman Program
The Legal Center
455 Sherman Street, Suite 130
Denver, CO 80203-4403
Phone: (800) 288-1376

Connecticut Dept. of Social Services
25 Sigourney Street, 10th Flr.
Hartford, CT 06106-5033
Phone: (860) 424-5200

Delaware Div. of Services for Aging &
Adults
1901 North Dupont Highway
Main Admin. Bldg. Annex
New Castle, DE 19720
Phone: (302) 577-4791

AARP Foundation
Legal Counsel for the Elderly
601 E Street, N.W., A4-330
Washington, DC 20049
Phone: (202) 434-2140

Florida State LTC Ombudsman Council
600 South Calhoun St., Suite 270
Tallahassee, FL 32301
Phone: (888) 831-0404

Georgia Division of Aging Services
2 Peachtree Street, NW
Suite 36-233
Atlanta, GA 30303-3142
Phone: (888) 454-5826

Hawaii Executive Office on Aging
250 South Hotel Street, Suite 109
Honolulu, HI 96865
Phone: (808) 586-0100

State Licensure & Cert. Programs

Colorado Dept of Health
Health Facilities Division
4300 Cherry Creek Dr. South
Denver, CO 80222-1530
Phone: (303) 692-2819

Connecticut Health Systems Regulation Div.
CT Dept of Public Health
410 Capital Ave. MS#12HSR
Hartford, CT 06134-0308
Phone: (860) 509-7400

Delaware Health Facilities Licensing & Cert.
Three Mill Rd. Suite 308
Wilmington, DE 19806-2114
Phone: (302) 577-6666

Department of Health
Licensing Regulation Administration
825 North Capitol Street, NE, Room 2264
Washington, DC 20002
Phone: (202) 442-4747

Florida Agency for Health Care Adm.
Division of Health Quality Assur.
2727 Mahan Drive, Room 200
Tallahassee, FL 32308-5403
Phone: (850) 487-2527

Georgia Dept. of Human Resources
Office of Regulatory Services
2 Peachtree Street, NW, 21st Floor
Suite 21-325
Atlanta, GA 30303-3167
Phone: (404) 657-5700

Hawaii Department of Health
Office of Health Care Assurance
601 Kamokila Blvd., Room 395
Kapolei, HI 96707
Phone: (808) 586-4080

State Ombudsman Programs

Idaho Commission on Aging
P.O. Box 837203380 American
Terrace, Suite 120
Boise, ID 83720-0007
Phone: (877) 471-2777

Illinois Department on Aging
421 E. Capitol Ave., Suite
100Springfield, IL 62701-1789
Phone: (217) 785-3143

Indiana Div. Disabilities/Rehab Services
402 W. Washington St., Room W 454
Indianapolis, IN 46207-7083Phone:
(800) 545-7763

Iowa Department of Elder
AffairsClements Building
200 10th Street
Des Moines, IA 50309-3609
Phone: (515) 242-3327

Kansas Office of the State LTC
Ombudsman
610 SW 10th Street, 2nd Flr.
Topeka, KS 66612-1616
Phone: (785) 296-3017 KY

Kentucky State Ombudsman Program
Office of Aging Services, 5W-A
275 E. Main Street
Frankfort, KY 40621
Phone: (800) 372-2991

Louisiana State LTC Program
412 N. 4th Street, 3rd Floor
Baton Rouge, LA 70802
Phone: (225) 342-1700

State Licensure & Cert. Programs

Idaho Bureau of Facility Standards
PO Box 83720
Boise, ID 83720-0036
Phone: (208) 364-1864

Illinois Office of Health Care Regulation
Illinois Dept. of Public Health
525 W. Jefferson, 5th Floor
Springfield, IL 62761
Phone: (217) 782-2913

Indiana HealthCare Regulatory
Services Commission
Indiana State Dept. of Health
2 North Meridian Street, Section 5A
Indianapolis, IN 46204
Phone: (317) 233-7022

Division of Health Facilities
Iowa Dept. of Inspections & Appeals
Lucas State Office Building, 3rd Floor
Des Moines, IA 50319-0083
Phone: (515) 281-4125

Kansas Dept. Health & Envrnmnt.
Health Facility Regulation
Bureau of Adult & Child Care
900 SW Jackson, Suite 1001
Topeka, KS 66612-1290
Phone: (785) 296-1260

Kentucky Office of Inspector General
Cabinet of Health Services
275 East Main Street
Frankfort, KY 40621-0001
Phone: (502) 564-2888

Louisiana Dept. of Health & Hospitals
Health Standards Section
P.O. Box 3767
Baton Rouge, LA 70821-3767
Phone: (225) 342-0415

State Ombudsman Programs

Maine State LTC Ombudsman Prog.
1 Weston CourtAugusta, ME 04332
Phone: (207) 621-1079

Maryland Department of Aging
301 W. Preston Street, Room 1007
Baltimore, MD 21201
Phone: (410) 767-1100

Massachusets Exec Office of Elder Affairs
1 Ashburton Place
5th Floor
Boston, MA 02108-1518
Phone: (617) 727-7750

Michigan Citizens for Better Care
4750 Woodward Avenue, Suite 410
Detroit, MI 48201-1308
Phone: (313) 832-6387

Office of Ombudsman for Older
Minnesotans
121 East Seventh Place, Ste. 410
St. Paul, MN 55101
Phone: (800) 657-3591

Missouri Div. on Aging
615 Howerton Court
Jefferson City, MO 65102-1337
Phone: (573) 526-0727

Mississippi Div. of Aging/Adult Services
750 North State Street
Jackson, MS 39202
Phone: (601) 359-4929

State Licensure & Cert. Programs

Maine Dept. of Human Services
Bureau of Medical Services
11 State House Station
35 Anthony Avenue
Augusta, ME 04333-0011
Phone: (207) 642-5443

Maryland Dept. of Health & Men. Hygiene
Licensing & Cert. Administration
55 Wade Avenue
Catonsville, MD 21228
Phone: (410) 402-8000

Massachusets Dept. of Public Health
Division Health Care Quality
10 West Street, 5th Floor
Boston, MA 02111
Phone: (617) 753-8100

Michigan Dept. of Consumer & Ind. Serv.
Div. of Health Fac. Lic. & Cert.
P.O. Box 30664
Lansing, MI 48909
Phone: (517) 241-2626

Minnesota - FPC/MDH
P.O. Box 64900
St. Paul, MN 55164-0900
Phone: (651) 215-8715

Missouri Department of Health
Bureau of Health Facility Regulation
PO Box 570
Jefferson City, MO 65102-0570
Phone: (537) 751-6302

Health Facilities Licensure & Cert.
Mississippi Department of Health
PO Box 1700
Jackson, MS 39215-1700
Phone: (601) 576-7300

State Ombudsman Programs

Senior & LTC Division
Montana Dept. of Health Serv.
P.O. Box 4210
Helena, MT 59604-4210
Phone: (800) 551-3191

Nebraska Division of Aging Services
P.O. Box 95044
Lincoln, NE 68509-5044
Phone: (402) 471-2307

Nevada Division for Aging
445 Apple Street, #104
Reno, NV 89502
Phone: (775) 688-2964

New Hampshire State LTC Ombusdman
129 Pleasant Street
Concord, NH 03301-3857
Phone: (603) 271-4375

New Jersey Office of Ombudsman
P.O. Box 807
Trenton, NJ 08625-0807
Phone: (609) 943-4026

New Mexico State Agency on
Aging228 E. Palace Avenue
Santa Fe, NM 87501
Phone: (505) 827-7663

New York State Office for the Aging
2 Empire State Plaza
Agency Building #2
Albany, NY 12223-0001
Phone: (518) 474-0108

State Licensure & Cert. Programs

Montana Certification Bureau
Montana Dept. of Health
PO Box 202951
Helena, MT 59620
Phone: (406) 444-2037

Nebraska Dept. of Health & Human
Services
PO Box 95007
Lincoln, NE 68509-5007
Phone: (402) 471-0179

Nevada Bureau Licensure & Certification
1550 East College Pkwy., Ste. 158
Carson City, NV 89706
Phone: (702) 687-4475

New Hampshire Office of Program Support
Health Facilities Admin.
129 Pleasant Street, Brown Bldg.
Concord, NH 03301
Phone: (603) 271-4966

New Jersey State Dept. of Health
Div. of Long Term Care Systems
CN 367
Trenton, NJ 08625-0367
Phone: (609) 633-8977

New Mexico Department of Health
Bureau of Health Fac. Lic. & Cert.
525 Camino De Los Marquez,#2
Santa Fe, NM 87501
Phone: (505) 827-4200

New York State Department of Health
Office of Continuing Care
161 Delaware Ave.
Delmar, NY 12054
Phone: (518) 474-1004

State Ombudsman Programs

North Carolina Division of Aging
2101 Mail Service Center, Room 634
Raleigh, NC 27626
Phone: (919) 733-8395

North Dakota Long Term Care
Ombudsman
Aging Services Division
600 South 2nd St., Suite 1C
Bismarck, ND 58504
Phone: (800) 451-8693

Ohio Department of Aging
50 W Broad Street9th Floor
Columbus, OH 43215-5928
Phone: (614) 644-7922

Oklahoma State LTC Ombudsman
Aging Services Division
312 NE 28th Street
Oklahoma City, OK 73105
Phone: (405) 521-6734

Oregon Office of the LTC Ombudsman
3855 Wolverine, NE, Suite 6
Salem, OR 97305
Phone: (503) 378-6533

Pennsylvania Department of Aging
555 Walnut Street, 5th Floor
Harrisburg, PA 17111
Phone: (717) 783-7247

State LTC Ombudsman
Puerto Rico Governor's
Call Box 50063
Old San Juan Station
San Juan, PR 00902
Phone: (787) 725-1515

State Licensure & Cert. Programs

North Carolina Department of Human
Resources
PO Box 29530
Raleigh, NC 27626-0530
Phone: (919) 733-7461

North Dakota State Department of Health
Health Resources Section
600 E Blvd. Ave.
Bismarck, ND 58505-2352
Phone: (701) 328-2352

Ohio Dvsn. of Health Fac. Regulation
Ohio Dept. of Health
246 North High Street
Columbus, OH 43266-0118
Phone: (614) 466-7857

Oklahoma State Department of Health
1000 NE 10th Street
Oklahoma City, OK 73117-1299
Phone: (405) 271-4200

Oregon Dept. of Human Resources
Senior & Disabled Services
500 Summer St., 2nd Fl.
Salem, OR 97310-1015
Phone: (503) 945-6456

Pennsylvania Dept. of Health
Bureau of Quality Assurance
PO Box 90
Harrisburg, PA 17108
Phone: (717) 787-8015

State Ombudsman Programs

Rhode Island Alliance for Better Long Term Care
422 Post Road, Ste. 204
Warwick, RI 02888
Phone: (401) 785-3340

South Carolina Office of Health & Human Serv.
P.O. Box 8206
Columbia, SC 29202-8206
Phone: (800) 868-9095

South Dakota Office of Adult Services & Aging
Department of Social Services
700 Governors Drive
Pierre, SD 57501-2291
Phone: (605) 773-3656

Tennessee Commission on Aging & Disability
Andrew Jackson Bldg.
7500 Deaderick St., 9th Flr.
Nashville, TN 37243-0860
Phone: (615) 741-2056

Texas Department on Aging
4900 N. Lamar Blvd. 4th Floor
Austin, TX 78711
Phone: (800) 252-2412

Utah Div of Aging & Adult Services
Department of Human Services
120 North 200 West, Room 401
Salt Lake City, UT 84103-0500
Phone: (801) 538-3924

State LTC Ombudsman
Vermont Legal Aid, Inc.
P.O. Box 1367
Burlington, VT 05402
Phone: (802) 863-5620

State Licensure & Cert. Programs

Div. of Facilities Regulation
Rhode Island Dept. of Health
3 Capitol Hill
Providence, RI 02908-5097
Phone: (401) 277-2566

S. Carolina Dept. of Health & Env. Control
Bureau of Certification
2600 Bull Street
Columbia, SC 29201-1708
Phone: (803) 737-7205

Office of Health Care Facilities
Health Systems Development and Reg.
615 E/ 4th St.
Pierre, SD 57501-5070
Phone: (605) 773-3356

Tennessee Dept. of Health
Health Care Facilities
425 5th Avenue North
Nashville, TN 37247-0508
Phone: (615) 741-7221

Long Term Care - Regulatory
Texas Dept. of Human Services
701 W 51st
Austin, TX 78714-9030
Phone: (512) 834-6696

Utah Bureau of Medicare/Medicaid
Program Certification
Div. of Health Systems Improvement
PO Box 16990
Salt Lake City, UT 84114-2905
Phone: (801) 538-6559

Vermont Dept. of Aging & Disabilities
Licensing & Protection Divis.
103 South Main Street
Waterbury, VT 05671-2306
Phone: (802) 241-2345

State Ombudsman Programs

Virginia Assoc. Area Agencies on Aging
530 East Main Street Suite 428
Richmond, VA 23219
Phone: (804) 644-2804

South King County Multi-Service Center
1200 South 336th Street
Federal Way, WA 98093-7452
Phone: (253) 838-6810

West Virginia Bureau of Senior Services
1900 Kanawha Blvd. East
Holly Grove Bldg., #1
Charleston, WV 25302
Phone: (304) 558-3317

Wisconsin Board on Aging & Long
Term Care
214 North Hamilton Street
Madison, WI 53703-2118
Phone: (800) 815-0015

Wyoming Senior Citizens Inc.
756 Gilchrist
Wheatland, WY 82201
Phone: (307) 322-5553

State Licensure & Cert. Programs

Virginia Department of Health
Office Health Facilities Reg.
3600 W. Broad, Suite 216
Richmond, VA 23230
Phone: (804) 367-2102

Washington Department of Social &
Health Services
Residential Care Services
PO Box 45600
Olympia, WA 98504-5600
Phone: (360) 493-2560

West Virginia Department of Health
Office of Hlth. Facility Lic.
350 Capitol St., Room 206
Charleston, WV 25301-3718
Phone: (304) 558-0050

Wisconsin Dept. of Health & Family
Services
PO Box 2969
Madison, WI 53701-2969
Phone: (608) 267-7185

Wyoming Health Facilities Program
Office of Health Quality
2020 Carey Ave., 8th Floor
Cheyenne, WY 82002
Phone: (307) 777-7123

Federal Licensing & Certification Agency
Centers for Medicare and Medicaid Services
CMSO/SBG/BNHCCS/NHB
7500 Security Boulevard
Baltimore, MD 21244-1850
Phone: (410) 786-3033

Index

Administration on Aging, 116
Advocacy, 1-3, 5, 17-19, 36-37,
  72, 96-97, 106-108, 116-118
  citizen groups, 115-116
  informal, 108-109
  litigation, 115
  ombudsman program and, 113-
    114
  quality of life and, 96-105
  reporting neglect and abuse, 115
  requesting a meeting and, 110-
    111
  resident and family councils, 112
  state licensing and certification
    offices, 114
  submitting a complaint, 111-112
Alzheimer's disease, 33
American Association of Homes
  and Services for the Aging
  (AAHSA,) 89
American Health Care Association
  (AHCA,) 89
Assessment, 6, 16, 38-41, 48, 85-
  86, 99-100, 101-102;
  case example, 50-57
Avoiding Chemical Restraint Use,
  90
Avoiding Physical Restraint Use, 90

Bedrails, 74,76
Behavioral symptoms, 73-74, 84-88

Carboni, Judith, 12, 15
Care planning, 6, 16, 38, 41-49,
  100, 102
  case example of, 20-22, 50-57
  right to participation in, 27-28

Care planning conferences, 43-47,
  69
Center for Medicare and Medicaid
  Services, 54
Certified Nursing Assistants (CNA's,)
  4, 55, 124
Citizen advocacy groups, 66, 68,
  72, 89, 115, 129, 149
Contractures, 68-70

Dehydration, 62-63
Delirium, 78
Dementing illnesses, 84
Depression, 80-81

Everyone Win! Program, 90

Family council, 34, 65, 70, 71, 112,
  141, 142

Hawes, Catherine, 14
Hygiene, 65-66

Improving the Quality of Care in
  Nursing Homes, 4
Incontinence, 61-62
Independence, 70-71
Individualized care, 8-14, 57, 87
  agitation and, 94-95
  assessment and care planning, 16
  life support measures and, 95
  postural needs and, 92
  quality of care, 14-15, 17-19
  quality of life, 15, 96-99
  resident function and, 91
  resident wandering and, 93-94
  safe environment and, 92-93

More Books With *IMPACT*

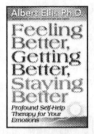
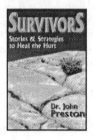
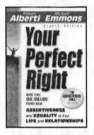
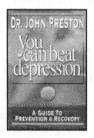

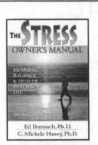
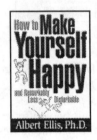
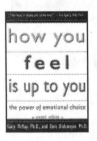
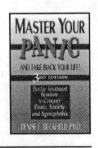